Preparing Pregnancy

for

New Parent

Everything you need to know for a healthy and confident pregnancy

Carmen R. Brown

TABLE OF CONTENT

Introduction

Welcome Message

Welcome to the exciting journey of pregnancy! Whether this is your first time becoming a parent or you're expanding your family, this book is here to be your trusted companion throughout the entire process. Pregnancy is a time filled with joy, anticipation, and a myriad of questions. Our goal is to provide you with the knowledge and support you need to navigate this incredible period with confidence and ease.

From the moment you start planning for pregnancy to the day you bring your baby home, this book covers every stage. We understand that each pregnancy is unique, and while there's no one-size-fits-all guide, we've compiled a comprehensive resource that addresses common experiences and concerns. Our hope is that by reading this book, you'll feel more prepared for the changes and milestones ahead, equipped with practical advice and reassured by the shared experiences of others.

Purpose of the Book

The purpose of this book is multifaceted. We aim to inform, support, and empower you during your pregnancy journey. Here's how we hope to achieve that:

1. **Inform**: Providing accurate and up-to-date information about pregnancy, childbirth, and early parenthood is our primary goal. Pregnancy can bring about significant physical, emotional, and mental changes, and understanding these changes can help alleviate anxiety and prepare you for what's to come. From the biological aspects of conception to the various stages of fetal development, we strive to offer clear, detailed explanations that will increase your understanding and confidence.

2. **Support**: Beyond providing information, we offer practical advice and tips for managing the various aspects of pregnancy. This includes nutrition and exercise guidelines, dealing with common pregnancy symptoms, preparing for labor and delivery, and understanding postpartum recovery. We also include advice on how to build a supportive network, both in terms of healthcare professionals and personal relationships.

3. **Empower**: We encourage you to make informed decisions about your pregnancy and childbirth. This involves discussing topics such as birth plans, pain management options, and the importance of advocating for yourself in healthcare settings. By presenting various options and considerations, we hope to empower you to choose what feels best for you and your baby.

4. **Reassure**: Addressing common concerns and questions that many expectant parents have is a key aspect of this book. Pregnancy can be a time of uncertainty, and we want you to know that you are not alone. The feelings and experiences you're having are shared by many, and there are answers and support available for the challenges you may face.

5. **Connect**: Highlighting the importance of building a support network, including healthcare providers, family, and friends, is crucial. Having a solid support system can make a significant difference in your pregnancy experience. This book provides guidance on how to build and maintain these connections, ensuring you have the help and encouragement you need along the way.

Pregnancy is a time of significant change, and with change often comes uncertainty. This book is here to provide clarity and comfort, helping you to enjoy the journey and cherish the moments.

This book is structured to be a comprehensive guide that you can refer to at any point during your pregnancy. Here are some tips on how to make the most of it:

1. **Read Chronologically**: While you can certainly jump to any section that interests you, reading the book from start to finish will provide a sequential understanding of pregnancy. Each chapter builds on the previous one, offering a complete picture of what to expect during each trimester and beyond. This approach will give you a holistic view of the journey ahead and help you prepare step by step.

2. **Use as a Reference Guide**: If you have specific questions or concerns, use the table of contents or index to find relevant sections quickly. Whether you're dealing with morning sickness, wondering about prenatal tests, or preparing for labor, you'll find detailed information and advice in the corresponding chapters. This makes the book a handy reference tool that you can consult whenever a question or concern arises.

3. **Take Notes**: Pregnancy is a personal experience, and what works for one person might not work for another. As you read, take notes on tips and advice

that resonate with you. You might also jot down questions to discuss with your healthcare provider during your prenatal visits. Keeping a journal alongside this book can be a helpful way to track your thoughts, feelings, and questions as you progress through your pregnancy.

4. **Engage with Exercises and Checklists**: Throughout the book, you'll find various exercises, checklists, and templates designed to help you plan and prepare. Engage with these tools to organize your thoughts and track your progress. For example, a birth plan template can help you outline your preferences for labor and delivery, while checklists can ensure you don't forget important tasks as your due date approaches.

5. **Join the Community**: At the end of the book, we've included a section on resources and support, including recommended books, websites, and support groups. Connecting with others who are going through similar experiences can provide additional support and encouragement. Whether it's through online forums, local parenting groups, or prenatal classes, building a community can make a big difference in your pregnancy experience.

6. **Stay Informed**: Pregnancy research is continually evolving, and while this book provides a comprehensive overview, it's essential to stay

informed about new developments. Regularly check in with your healthcare provider and consult reputable sources for the latest information. This ongoing learning will help you feel more confident and capable throughout your pregnancy.

7. **Trust Yourself**: While we provide a wealth of information and advice, remember that you know your body and your needs best. Use this book as a guide, but trust your instincts and make choices that feel right for you and your baby. Every pregnancy is unique, and what matters most is that you feel supported and empowered in your decisions.

Making the Most of Your Pregnancy Journey

Your pregnancy journey is a unique and personal experience, and we want this book to be a supportive and valuable resource every step of the way. Here are some final tips on how to make the most of it:

- **Stay Positive**: Pregnancy can be overwhelming, but try to focus on the positive aspects. Celebrate the milestones, no matter how small, and take time to appreciate the incredible process your body is going through. A positive mindset can make a big difference in how you experience pregnancy.
- **Stay Connected**: Share your experiences and feelings with your partner, family, and friends.

Building a support network can provide emotional and practical support, making the journey smoother. Don't hesitate to reach out to others for help or companionship.

- **Stay Healthy**: Follow the guidelines and advice provided in the book on nutrition, exercise, and prenatal care. Taking care of your physical health will positively impact your emotional and mental well-being. Regular checkups, a balanced diet, and staying active are key components of a healthy pregnancy.

- **Stay Flexible**: Pregnancy rarely goes exactly as planned, so stay flexible and open to changes. Adapt as needed and seek help when you encounter challenges. Whether it's adjusting your birth plan or seeking support for unexpected symptoms, being adaptable will help you navigate the ups and downs of pregnancy.

- **Stay Informed**: Continue learning and asking questions throughout your pregnancy. The more you know, the more empowered you'll feel to make the best decisions for yourself and your baby. Knowledge is power, and staying informed will help you feel more in control.

We hope this book will be a constant companion, offering the information, reassurance, and support you need to navigate your pregnancy with confidence and joy. Congratulations on your pregnancy, and we wish you all the best on this incredible journey!

Chapter 1: Preconception Planning

Importance of Preconception Health

Embarking on the journey to parenthood is an exciting and transformative time, but it also comes with its own set of challenges and responsibilities. One of the most crucial steps in this journey is ensuring that you are in the best possible health before you conceive. Preconception health refers to the state of your health before becoming pregnant and plays a significant role in the health and development of your future baby.

Why Preconception Health Matters

Preconception health is important for several reasons:

1. **Reducing Risks for Mother and Baby**: Proper preconception health can reduce the risk of complications during pregnancy and childbirth, such as preeclampsia, gestational diabetes, and preterm birth. It also helps in ensuring the baby's healthy development.

2. **Enhancing Fertility**: A healthy lifestyle, including a balanced diet, regular exercise, and avoiding harmful substances, can improve fertility for both partners. It increases the chances of conceiving and sustaining a healthy pregnancy.

3. **Early Detection and Management of Health Issues**: Addressing any pre-existing health conditions or risks before pregnancy can prevent complications. Conditions like diabetes, high blood pressure, and thyroid disorders can be managed more effectively with early intervention.
4. **Genetic Health**: Understanding and addressing genetic risks before pregnancy can prevent the transmission of genetic disorders. Genetic screening can identify potential issues that can be managed with appropriate medical intervention.
5. **Emotional and Mental Preparedness**: Being in good physical health often correlates with better emotional and mental well-being, which is crucial during the demanding phases of pregnancy and early parenthood.

Taking steps to improve your preconception health is a proactive approach to ensuring a smoother pregnancy and a healthier baby. This chapter will guide you through the various aspects of preconception health, starting with preconception counseling.

Preconception Counseling

Preconception counseling is a vital step for anyone planning to become pregnant. It involves meeting with a healthcare provider to discuss your health, lifestyle, and any factors that might affect your pregnancy. This counseling session helps in identifying and mitigating risks, providing education, and planning for a healthy pregnancy.

What to Expect During Preconception Counseling

During a preconception counseling session, your healthcare provider will review several aspects of your health and lifestyle:

1. **Personal Medical History**: Your provider will ask about any chronic health conditions you may have, such as epilepsy, diabetes, high blood pressure, anemia, or allergies. It's important to manage these conditions effectively before conception to reduce risks during pregnancy.
2. **Current Medications**: You will need to discuss any medications you are currently taking, including over-the-counter drugs and supplements. Some medications can affect fertility or may not be safe during pregnancy, and your provider can suggest safer alternatives if necessary.
3. **Previous Surgeries and Past Pregnancies**: Any previous surgeries, especially those involving the reproductive system, will be reviewed. If you've had past pregnancies, including any complications such as miscarriage or preterm labor, these will be

discussed to plan for a healthier outcome in future pregnancies.

4. **Family Medical History**: An assessment of both maternal and paternal medical history helps identify any genetic or hereditary conditions that might affect your pregnancy or your baby's health. Conditions like high blood pressure, diabetes, and birth defects will be noted.

5. **Genetic Screening**: Genetic counseling and screening tests may be recommended based on your medical and family history. This can help identify the risk of inherited genetic disorders such as sickle cell anemia, Tay-Sachs disease, or cystic fibrosis.

6. **Vaccine Status**: Your provider will ensure that you are up-to-date on vaccines that are crucial for a healthy pregnancy, such as rubella (German measles) and varicella (chickenpox). If you lack immunity to these diseases, you should get vaccinated at least a month before trying to conceive.

7. **Lifestyle Factors**: Discussions will include your diet, exercise habits, substance use (such as smoking or alcohol), and any other lifestyle factors that could impact your pregnancy. Your provider will offer guidance on making healthy changes to optimize your fertility and pregnancy outcomes.

8. **Mental Health**: Mental and emotional health is equally important. Your provider may screen for

depression, anxiety, and other mental health issues. They can offer resources and support to ensure you are emotionally prepared for pregnancy.

Benefits of Preconception Counseling

Preconception counseling offers numerous benefits:

1. **Personalized Care**: The counseling session provides tailored advice and interventions based on your individual health and lifestyle. This personalized approach ensures that specific risks are addressed effectively.
2. **Preventive Health**: Early identification and management of potential health issues can prevent complications during pregnancy. For example, controlling blood sugar levels in women with diabetes can reduce the risk of birth defects.
3. **Informed Decision-Making**: Counseling equips you with the knowledge needed to make informed decisions about your health and pregnancy. Understanding the risks and benefits of various interventions helps you take proactive steps for a healthy pregnancy.
4. **Peace of Mind**: Knowing that you have taken steps to optimize your health before pregnancy can provide peace of mind and reduce anxiety. Being

well-prepared allows you to focus on enjoying your pregnancy journey.

5. **Improved Outcomes**: Studies have shown that preconception care improves pregnancy outcomes. Women who receive preconception counseling are more likely to have healthy pregnancies and deliver healthy babies.

Medical and Family History

Understanding your medical and family history is a cornerstone of preconception planning. It provides valuable insights into potential risks and helps in formulating a comprehensive plan for a healthy pregnancy.

Personal Medical History

Your personal medical history includes any chronic conditions, past surgeries, and previous pregnancies. Here are some key aspects to consider:

1. **Chronic Conditions**: Conditions like diabetes, hypertension, thyroid disorders, epilepsy, and asthma need to be well-controlled before pregnancy. Poorly managed conditions can lead to complications such as preeclampsia, preterm birth, and congenital anomalies.

2. **Current Medications**: Some medications can affect fertility or may not be safe during pregnancy. Your healthcare provider will review your medications and suggest safer alternatives if needed. Never stop taking prescribed medication without consulting your provider.

3. **Previous Surgeries**: Surgeries, especially those involving the reproductive organs, can impact fertility and pregnancy. Discuss any previous surgeries with your provider to understand their implications.

4. **Past Pregnancies**: If you've had previous pregnancies, including any complications such as miscarriage, preterm labor, or gestational diabetes, your provider will consider these factors in your preconception plan. Understanding past issues helps in planning for a healthier outcome in future pregnancies.

Family Medical History

Family medical history provides insights into genetic conditions and hereditary risks. Both maternal and paternal histories are important:

1. **Genetic Disorders**: Certain genetic disorders can be inherited, such as sickle cell anemia, cystic fibrosis, and Tay-Sachs disease. Understanding your family's

genetic history helps in assessing the risk of passing these conditions to your child.

2. **Chronic Conditions**: Conditions like diabetes, hypertension, and heart disease can have a genetic component. Knowing if these conditions are prevalent in your family can help in early monitoring and intervention.

3. **Birth Defects and Intellectual Disabilities**: If there are any birth defects or intellectual disabilities in your family, discuss these with your healthcare provider. Early screening and intervention can help manage these risks.

Importance of Accurate Information

Providing accurate and detailed information about your medical and family history is crucial. It allows your healthcare provider to:

1. **Identify Risks**: Early identification of potential risks enables timely interventions to prevent complications.

2. **Plan for Screening**: Genetic screening and other tests can be planned based on your history, ensuring that any issues are detected early.

3. **Provide Tailored Advice**: Personalized recommendations can be made to optimize your health and pregnancy outcomes.

4. **Manage Chronic Conditions**: Effective management of chronic conditions reduces the risk of complications during pregnancy.

Genetic Screening

Genetic screening is an essential part of preconception planning. It involves testing for certain genetic disorders that could be passed on to your child. Understanding the risk of these disorders allows you to make informed decisions about your pregnancy and take steps to manage potential issues.

What is Genetic Screening?

Genetic screening tests analyze your DNA to identify mutations or changes in specific genes that can cause genetic disorders. These tests can be performed on a blood sample or saliva and provide information about your risk of having a child with a genetic condition.

Common Genetic Disorders

Some common genetic disorders that can be screened for include:

1. **Cystic Fibrosis**: A disorder that affects the respiratory and digestive systems. It is caused by mutations in the CFTR gene.
2. **Sickle Cell Anemia**: A blood disorder that causes red blood cells to become misshapen and break down. It is caused by a mutation in the HBB gene.
3. **Tay-Sachs Disease**: A disorder that destroys nerve cells in the brain and spinal cord. It is caused by mutations in the HEXA gene.
4. **Thalassemia**: A blood disorder that causes the body to make an abnormal form of hemoglobin. It is caused by mutations in the HBA1, HBA2, or HBB genes.
5. **Fragile X Syndrome**: A genetic condition that causes intellectual disability and developmental delays. It is caused by mutations in the FMR1 gene.

Who Should Consider Genetic Screening?

Genetic screening is recommended for:

1. **Couples with a Family History of Genetic Disorders**: If you or your partner have a family history of genetic conditions, screening can help assess the risk of passing these conditions to your child.
2. **Couples from High-Risk Ethnic Backgrounds**: Certain genetic disorders are more common in

specific ethnic groups. For example, Tay-Sachs disease is more prevalent in individuals of Ashkenazi Jewish descent.

3. **Couples with Previous Pregnancy Complications**: If you've had a previous pregnancy affected by a genetic disorder or birth defect, genetic screening can help identify any underlying genetic causes.

4. **All Couples Planning a Pregnancy**: Even if you don't have a known family history of genetic disorders, genetic screening can provide valuable information about your risk.

Types of Genetic Screening Tests

1. **Carrier Screening**: Tests to determine if you carry a gene for a recessive genetic disorder. Carriers typically do not show symptoms but can pass the gene to their children.

2. **Preimplantation Genetic Testing (PGT)**: Used in conjunction with in vitro fertilization (IVF) to test embryos for genetic disorders before implantation.

3. **Prenatal Screening**: Tests performed during pregnancy to detect genetic conditions in the fetus. These include non-invasive prenatal testing (NIPT), chorionic villus sampling (CVS), and amniocentesis.

Benefits of Genetic Screening

1. **Informed Decision-Making**: Knowing your genetic risk allows you to make informed decisions about your pregnancy, including whether to pursue additional testing or consider reproductive options such as IVF with PGT.
2. **Early Intervention**: Early identification of genetic disorders enables early intervention and management, improving outcomes for affected children.
3. **Peace of Mind**: Understanding your genetic risk can provide peace of mind and reduce anxiety about potential genetic conditions.

Limitations of Genetic Screening

1. **Not All Conditions Can Be Detected**: Genetic screening tests do not detect all genetic disorders. Some conditions may go undetected even with comprehensive screening.
2. **Uncertainty**: Some test results may be inconclusive or indicate an increased risk without providing a definitive diagnosis. This can lead to uncertainty and anxiety.
3. **Ethical Considerations**: Genetic screening raises ethical considerations, such as the potential for discrimination based on genetic information and the decision-making process regarding affected pregnancies.

Vaccinations play a crucial role in preconception planning by protecting both the mother and baby from preventable diseases. Ensuring that you are up-to-date on essential vaccinations before becoming pregnant can prevent serious complications and safeguard your health and your baby's development.

Key Vaccinations Before Pregnancy

1. **Rubella (German Measles)**
   - **Importance**: Rubella infection during pregnancy can cause serious birth defects known as congenital rubella syndrome, leading to heart problems, developmental delays, and hearing impairments.
   - **Vaccination**: The MMR (measles, mumps, rubella) vaccine is recommended for women who are not immune. It is important to receive this vaccine at least one month before trying to conceive, as it is a live vaccine and not recommended during pregnancy.
2. **Varicella (Chickenpox)**
   - **Importance**: Varicella infection during pregnancy can lead to severe complications for both the mother and the baby, including congenital varicella syndrome and neonatal varicella.

- **Vaccination**: The varicella vaccine is recommended for women who have not had chickenpox or the vaccine. Like the MMR vaccine, it should be administered at least one month before conception.

3. **Hepatitis B**
   - **Importance**: Hepatitis B can be transmitted from mother to baby during childbirth, leading to chronic infection and liver disease in the child.
   - **Vaccination**: The hepatitis B vaccine is recommended for women who are at risk of infection, such as those with multiple sexual partners, healthcare workers, or women with hepatitis B-positive partners.

4. **Influenza (Flu)**
   - **Importance**: Influenza can cause severe illness in pregnant women and increase the risk of preterm labor and delivery. The flu vaccine helps protect both the mother and baby.
   - **Vaccination**: The flu vaccine is safe and recommended during any trimester of pregnancy. It is also recommended before pregnancy to ensure immunity during flu season.

5. **Tetanus, Diphtheria, and Pertussis (Tdap)**
   - **Importance**: Pertussis (whooping cough) can be life-threatening for newborns. Vaccination during

pregnancy helps protect the baby until they can receive their own vaccines.

- **Vaccination**: The Tdap vaccine is recommended during the third trimester of each pregnancy. It is also advisable to ensure that you are up-to-date with your tetanus and diphtheria vaccinations before pregnancy.

Vaccine Safety and Timing

1. **Live Vaccines**: Live vaccines, such as MMR and varicella, should be administered at least one month before trying to conceive. These vaccines are not recommended during pregnancy due to the potential risk to the developing fetus.
2. **Inactivated Vaccines**: Inactivated vaccines, such as the flu and Tdap vaccines, are safe to receive during pregnancy. They help protect both the mother and baby from preventable diseases.
3. **Consult Your Healthcare Provider**: Before receiving any vaccinations, consult with your healthcare provider to ensure you are up-to-date and to discuss the best timing for any needed vaccines.

Addressing Vaccine Concerns

Some individuals may have concerns about vaccines, including their safety and potential side effects. It is important to discuss any concerns with your healthcare provider, who can provide evidence-based information and address any misconceptions. Vaccines are rigorously tested for safety and effectiveness and are a crucial part of preconception and prenatal care.

Maintaining Immunity During Pregnancy

Ensuring you are up-to-date on vaccinations before pregnancy helps protect you and your baby from preventable diseases. It also contributes to herd immunity, reducing the spread of infectious diseases within the community. Maintaining a healthy immune system through vaccination is an essential aspect of preconception planning and overall reproductive health.

By focusing on preconception health, engaging in preconception counseling, understanding medical and family history, undergoing genetic screening, and ensuring you are up-to-date on essential vaccinations, you are taking proactive steps toward a healthy pregnancy and a healthy baby. These measures help reduce risks, enhance fertility, and provide peace of mind as you embark on your journey to parenthood.

Chapter 2: Healthy Lifestyle Changes

Preparing for pregnancy involves adopting a healthy lifestyle to ensure the best possible start for both you and your baby. This chapter will cover essential aspects of maintaining a healthy lifestyle, including nutrition and diet, exercise and fitness, avoiding harmful substances, managing stress and mental health, and the importance of sleep.

Nutrition and Diet

A balanced diet is crucial for overall health and fertility. Good nutrition before and during pregnancy can help you achieve and maintain a healthy weight, enhance fertility, and support the development of your baby. Here are some key points to consider:

Balanced Diet: Aim to consume a variety of foods from all the major food groups. This includes fruits, vegetables, whole grains, lean proteins, and dairy. Each of these groups provides essential nutrients that play a critical role in your health and your baby's development.

Fruits and Vegetables: These are rich in vitamins, minerals, and fiber. Aim to fill half your plate with fruits and vegetables at each meal. They are particularly high in folate (a natural form of folic acid) and other important vitamins like vitamin C.

Whole Grains: Foods such as whole wheat bread, brown rice, and quinoa provide fiber, which is essential for maintaining healthy digestion. Whole grains also contain important nutrients like iron, B vitamins, and magnesium.

Lean Proteins: Include a variety of protein sources such as poultry, fish, beans, and legumes. Protein is crucial for the growth and repair of tissues. Fish, in particular, provides omega-3 fatty acids, which are beneficial for brain development.

Dairy: Dairy products like milk, cheese, and yogurt provide calcium, vitamin D, and other essential nutrients that are important for bone health. If you are lactose intolerant or vegan, look for fortified plant-based alternatives.

Folic Acid: Start taking a folic acid supplement of at least 400 micrograms daily, ideally three months before conception. Folic acid helps prevent neural tube defects, which are serious birth defects of the brain and spine.

Hydration: Staying hydrated is important for maintaining healthy bodily functions. Aim to drink at least eight glasses of water a day. Limit sugary drinks and caffeine.

Caffeine: High caffeine intake is linked to an increased risk of miscarriage. Limit your caffeine intake to no more than 200 milligrams per day, which is roughly equivalent to one 12-ounce cup of coffee.

Alcohol: Avoid alcohol entirely when trying to conceive and during pregnancy. Alcohol can affect fertility and cause fetal alcohol spectrum disorders (FASD), which can result in lifelong physical, behavioral, and intellectual disabilities.

Vitamins and Supplements: In addition to folic acid, consider taking a prenatal vitamin that includes iron, calcium, and DHA. These nutrients are vital for a healthy pregnancy.

Eating Habits: Develop healthy eating habits by planning balanced meals and snacks. Eating smaller, frequent meals can help manage nausea and maintain energy levels throughout the day.

Avoid Processed Foods: Highly processed foods are often high in unhealthy fats, sugars, and salt. Opt for fresh, whole foods whenever possible.

Adopting these nutritional practices can improve your overall health and create a favorable environment for conception and a healthy pregnancy.

Regular physical activity is beneficial for both your fertility and your overall health. Exercise can help you maintain a healthy weight, reduce stress, and improve your mood. Here are some guidelines for incorporating exercise into your pregnancy preparation:

Benefits of Exercise: Engaging in regular exercise can enhance your fertility by improving blood circulation, balancing hormones, and reducing stress. Exercise also strengthens muscles, improves cardiovascular health, and increases flexibility, which can all be beneficial during pregnancy and childbirth.

Types of Exercise: Aim for a combination of aerobic exercises, strength training, and flexibility exercises. Aerobic exercises like walking, swimming, and cycling improve cardiovascular health. Strength training exercises such as weight lifting or bodyweight exercises build muscle strength. Flexibility exercises like yoga and stretching improve your range of motion and help prevent injury.

Moderate Intensity: Aim for at least 150 minutes of moderate-intensity aerobic activity each week. Moderate-intensity means you are working hard enough to raise your heart rate and break a sweat, but you can still talk comfortably.

Strength Training: Incorporate strength training exercises at least two days a week. Focus on major muscle groups, including legs, back, abdomen, chest, shoulders, and arms.

Flexibility and Balance: Yoga and stretching exercises can improve flexibility and balance, reduce stress, and help you stay relaxed. Prenatal yoga classes can be particularly beneficial, as they are designed to address the specific needs of pregnant women.

Stay Hydrated: Drink plenty of water before, during, and after exercise to stay hydrated.

Listen to Your Body: Pay attention to how your body feels during exercise. Avoid any activities that cause pain, dizziness, or shortness of breath. If you are new to exercise or have any health concerns, consult your healthcare provider before starting a new exercise routine.

Avoid High-Risk Activities: Avoid activities that have a high risk of injury, such as contact sports, horseback riding, or skiing. Also, avoid exercises that involve lying flat on your back after the first trimester, as this can reduce blood flow to the baby.

Exercise with a Partner: Exercising with your partner can be a great way to stay motivated and support each other's health goals.

By incorporating regular physical activity into your routine, you can improve your overall health and prepare your body for the demands of pregnancy and childbirth.

Avoiding Harmful Substances

Exposure to harmful substances can negatively impact your fertility and the health of your baby. It is essential to avoid these substances before and during pregnancy:

Tobacco: Smoking reduces fertility in both men and women and increases the risk of miscarriage, stillbirth, and premature birth. Even exposure to secondhand smoke can be harmful. Quitting smoking is one of the best things you can do for your health and the health of your baby. Seek support from your healthcare provider or a smoking cessation program if needed.

Alcohol: Alcohol can affect fertility and cause birth defects and developmental disorders. Avoid alcohol entirely when trying to conceive and during pregnancy.

Recreational Drugs: Illegal drugs such as marijuana, cocaine, and methamphetamines can cause serious health problems for both you and your baby. These substances can affect fertility, increase the risk of miscarriage, and lead to birth defects and developmental issues. Seek help from your healthcare provider if you need assistance quitting.

Caffeine: High caffeine intake is linked to an increased risk of miscarriage and may affect fertility. Limit your caffeine intake to no more than 200 milligrams per day, equivalent to one 12-ounce cup of coffee.

Environmental Toxins: Avoid exposure to harmful chemicals and toxins, such as pesticides, lead, and certain cleaning products. Use natural or non-toxic alternatives whenever possible. Avoid handling cat litter, which can contain toxoplasmosis, a parasite that can cause serious harm to your baby.

Medications: Review all medications you are taking with your healthcare provider to ensure they are safe for pregnancy. This includes prescription medications, over-the-counter drugs, and herbal supplements. Do not stop taking any prescribed medication without consulting your healthcare provider.

Radiation: Avoid unnecessary exposure to radiation, such as X-rays, especially during pregnancy. If you need an X-ray, inform your healthcare provider and the technician that you are trying to conceive or are pregnant.

By avoiding harmful substances, you can protect your fertility and create a safer environment for your baby's development.

Mental and emotional well-being are crucial aspects of preparing for pregnancy. Managing stress and maintaining good mental health can improve your overall well-being and increase your chances of conceiving:

Identify Stressors: Identify the sources of stress in your life and develop strategies to manage them. This may involve setting boundaries at work, seeking support from friends and family, or finding healthy ways to cope with stress.

Relaxation Techniques: Incorporate relaxation techniques into your daily routine. Techniques such as deep breathing, meditation, and progressive muscle relaxation can help reduce stress and promote a sense of calm.

Mindfulness: Practicing mindfulness involves staying present in the moment and being aware of your thoughts and feelings without judgment. Mindfulness techniques, such as mindful breathing and mindful walking, can help reduce stress and improve mental clarity.

Physical Activity: Regular exercise is a natural stress reliever. Physical activity releases endorphins, which are chemicals in the brain that act as natural painkillers and mood elevators.

Sleep: Ensure you are getting enough sleep, as sleep deprivation can increase stress levels and affect mental health. Establish a regular sleep routine and create a relaxing bedtime environment.

Social Support: Build a strong support network of friends, family, and healthcare providers. Having a support system can provide emotional and practical assistance during the preconception period and throughout pregnancy.

Counseling and Therapy: Consider seeking professional counseling or therapy if you are experiencing high levels of stress, anxiety, or depression. A mental health professional can help you develop coping strategies and provide support.

Hobbies and Interests: Engage in activities that you enjoy and that bring you joy. Hobbies and interests can provide a healthy distraction from stress and improve your overall well-being.

Healthy Relationships: Maintain healthy relationships with your partner, family, and friends. Open communication, mutual respect, and support are essential components of healthy relationships.

Positive Thinking: Practice positive thinking and focus on the aspects of your life that you are grateful for. Keeping a gratitude journal can help you cultivate a positive mindset.

By managing stress and prioritizing your mental health, you can create a positive environment for yourself and your baby.

Importance of Sleep

Adequate sleep is essential for overall health and well-being. Quality sleep is particularly important when preparing for pregnancy, as it affects your physical health, mental health, and fertility:

Sleep and Fertility: Studies have shown that poor sleep quality and insufficient sleep can negatively impact fertility. Sleep affects the regulation of hormones that play a crucial role in reproduction, such as melatonin and cortisol.

Sleep Hygiene: Establish good sleep hygiene practices to improve the quality of your sleep. This includes maintaining a regular sleep schedule, creating a relaxing bedtime routine, and creating a sleep-friendly environment.

Regular Sleep Schedule: Go to bed and wake up at the same time every day, even on weekends. Consistency helps regulate your body's internal clock and improves sleep quality.

Bedtime Routine: Develop a relaxing bedtime routine to signal to your body that it's time to wind down. This may include activities such as reading, taking a warm bath, or practicing relaxation techniques.

Sleep Environment: Create a comfortable and sleep-friendly environment in your bedroom. Ensure your mattress and pillows are supportive, keep the room cool and dark, and minimize noise and light.

Limit Screen Time: Avoid screens (such as phones, tablets, and computers) at least an hour before bedtime. The blue light emitted by screens can interfere with the production of melatonin, a hormone that regulates sleep.

Avoid Stimulants: Avoid consuming caffeine and nicotine close to bedtime, as these stimulants can interfere with sleep. Limit alcohol consumption, as it can disrupt sleep patterns.

Physical Activity: Engage in regular physical activity, but avoid vigorous exercise close to bedtime. Exercise can help you fall asleep faster and enjoy deeper sleep.

Diet: Be mindful of your diet and avoid heavy meals close to bedtime. Eating a light snack before bed can help prevent hunger and promote better sleep.

Relaxation Techniques: Practice relaxation techniques before bed to calm your mind and prepare your body for sleep. Techniques such as deep breathing, meditation, and progressive muscle relaxation can be effective.

Address Sleep Disorders: If you have difficulty falling asleep, staying asleep, or experience excessive daytime sleepiness, consult your healthcare provider. Sleep disorders such as insomnia or sleep apnea can affect your overall health and fertility.

By prioritizing sleep and adopting healthy sleep habits, you can improve your overall well-being and create a conducive environment for conception and a healthy pregnancy.

Preparing for pregnancy involves making healthy lifestyle changes that benefit both you and your baby. By focusing on nutrition and diet, exercise and fitness, avoiding harmful substances, managing stress and mental health, and prioritizing sleep, you can create a strong foundation for a healthy and confident pregnancy. Each of these aspects plays a crucial role in enhancing fertility, supporting a healthy pregnancy, and ensuring the well-being of both the mother and the baby. Embrace these changes as positive steps towards a healthier future and a joyful pregnancy journey.

Chapter 3: Fertility Awareness

Understanding and enhancing fertility is a crucial aspect of planning for pregnancy. This chapter will provide an in-depth look at the menstrual cycle, tracking ovulation, enhancing fertility for both partners, and addressing common fertility challenges.

Understanding the Menstrual Cycle

The menstrual cycle is a series of natural changes in hormone production and the structures of the uterus and ovaries of the female reproductive system that make pregnancy possible. Understanding the menstrual cycle is fundamental to fertility awareness.

Phases of the Menstrual Cycle

1. **Menstrual Phase (Days 1-5)**
   - This phase starts with the first day of menstruation and typically lasts for about five days.
   - The uterus sheds its lining, resulting in menstrual bleeding.
   - Hormone levels are low during this phase, particularly estrogen and progesterone.
2. **Follicular Phase (Days 1-13)**
   - Overlaps with the menstrual phase but continues until ovulation.

- The pituitary gland releases follicle-stimulating hormone (FSH), which stimulates the ovaries to produce several follicles, each containing an egg.
- Estrogen levels rise, leading to the thickening of the uterine lining in preparation for a possible pregnancy.

3. **Ovulation (Day 14)**
   - Typically occurs around the midpoint of the cycle but can vary.
   - A surge in luteinizing hormone (LH) triggers the release of a mature egg from one of the ovaries.
   - The egg travels down the fallopian tube, where it may meet sperm and become fertilized.

4. **Luteal Phase (Days 15-28)**
   - After ovulation, the ruptured follicle transforms into the corpus luteum, which secretes progesterone.
   - Progesterone maintains the thickened uterine lining.
   - If fertilization does not occur, the corpus luteum degenerates, leading to a drop in progesterone and the start of a new menstrual cycle.

Understanding these phases can help in identifying the fertile window, the time during the menstrual cycle when pregnancy is most likely to occur.

Tracking ovulation is essential for identifying the most fertile days in the menstrual cycle. There are several methods to track ovulation:

1. **Calendar Method**
   - This involves tracking the length of menstrual cycles over several months to predict ovulation.
   - Ovulation typically occurs around 14 days before the start of the next period.
   - This method is most effective for women with regular cycles.
2. **Basal Body Temperature (BBT) Charting**
   - BBT is the body's temperature at rest.
   - Slight increase in BBT (about 0.5 to 1 degree Fahrenheit) occurs after ovulation due to progesterone.
   - Track BBT daily before getting out of bed to identify the rise in temperature.
3. **Cervical Mucus Monitoring**
   - Cervical mucus changes throughout the menstrual cycle.
   - Around ovulation, cervical mucus becomes clear, stretchy, and slippery (like egg whites), indicating high fertility.

- Monitoring these changes can help pinpoint ovulation.

4. **Ovulation Predictor Kits (OPKs)**
   - OPKs detect the surge in LH that precedes ovulation.
   - Using OPKs around the expected ovulation period can help identify the best time for conception.

5. **Fertility Apps and Devices**
   - Various apps and devices are available that use algorithms to predict ovulation based on entered data like BBT, menstrual cycle length, and cervical mucus changes.
   - Some devices use sensors to provide real-time fertility insights.

By combining these methods, couples can increase their chances of accurately predicting ovulation and timing intercourse for conception.

Enhancing Fertility for Both Partners

Fertility is not solely dependent on the female partner. Both partners can take steps to enhance their fertility.

For Women

1. **Maintain a Healthy Diet**
   - A balanced diet rich in fruits, vegetables, whole grains, lean proteins, and healthy fats can improve overall health and fertility.
   - Specific nutrients like folic acid, iron, and omega-3 fatty acids are crucial for reproductive health.
2. **Exercise Regularly**
   - Regular, moderate exercise helps maintain a healthy weight and reduce stress, both of which are important for fertility.
   - Avoid excessive exercise, which can disrupt the menstrual cycle and ovulation.
3. **Maintain a Healthy Weight**
   - Both underweight and overweight women can experience irregular menstrual cycles and ovulation issues.
   - Achieving a healthy weight through diet and exercise can enhance fertility.
4. **Avoid Smoking and Alcohol**
   - Smoking and excessive alcohol consumption can negatively impact fertility and increase the risk of miscarriage.
   - Quitting smoking and limiting alcohol intake can improve reproductive health.

5. **Reduce Stress**
   - High stress levels can affect hormone balance and ovulation.
   - Practices like yoga, meditation, and mindfulness can help manage stress.
6. **Check Medication and Supplement Use**
   - Certain medications and supplements can affect fertility.
   - Consult a healthcare provider to ensure that any medication or supplement is safe for conception.

For Men

1. **Maintain a Healthy Diet**
   - A diet rich in antioxidants (like vitamins C and E), zinc, and selenium can improve sperm quality.
   - Healthy fats and adequate protein intake are also important for sperm production.
2. **Exercise Regularly**
   - Regular exercise can improve overall health and boost testosterone levels.
   - Avoid activities that overheat the testicles, like excessive cycling or using hot tubs, which can negatively impact sperm quality.
3. **Maintain a Healthy Weight**

- Being overweight or underweight can affect sperm count and quality.
- Achieving a healthy weight through diet and exercise can enhance fertility.

4. **Avoid Smoking and Excessive Alcohol**
   - Smoking and heavy drinking can reduce sperm count and motility.
   - Quitting smoking and moderating alcohol intake can improve sperm health.

5. **Reduce Exposure to Toxins**
   - Exposure to environmental toxins like pesticides, heavy metals, and chemicals can affect sperm quality.
   - Taking steps to reduce exposure, like using natural cleaning products and eating organic foods, can help.

6. **Manage Stress**
   - High stress levels can affect hormone balance and sperm production.
   - Practices like exercise, relaxation techniques, and hobbies can help manage stress.

7. **Check Medication and Supplement Use**
   - Certain medications and supplements can impact sperm production and quality.
   - Consult a healthcare provider to ensure that any medication or supplement is safe for conception.

Fertility challenges can affect both partners and may require medical intervention. Understanding these challenges can help in seeking appropriate treatment.

For Women

1. **Polycystic Ovary Syndrome (PCOS)**
   - PCOS is a common hormonal disorder that can cause irregular menstrual cycles and ovulation issues.
   - Symptoms include irregular periods, excessive hair growth, acne, and weight gain.
   - Treatment may include lifestyle changes, medication to regulate ovulation, and assisted reproductive technologies.
2. **Endometriosis**
   - Endometriosis occurs when tissue similar to the lining of the uterus grows outside the uterus, causing pain and fertility issues.
   - Symptoms include painful periods, pelvic pain, and pain during intercourse.
   - Treatment options include medication, surgery, and assisted reproductive technologies.

3. **Ovulation Disorders**
    - Various conditions can affect ovulation, including thyroid disorders, hyperprolactinemia, and premature ovarian failure.
    - Symptoms include irregular or absent menstrual periods.
    - Treatment may involve medication to induce ovulation or addressing underlying health conditions.

4. **Uterine or Cervical Abnormalities**
    - Structural issues with the uterus or cervix, such as fibroids, polyps, or congenital anomalies, can affect fertility.
    - Treatment options include surgery or assisted reproductive technologies.

5. **Tubal Factors**
    - Blocked or damaged fallopian tubes can prevent the egg and sperm from meeting.
    - Causes include pelvic inflammatory disease, previous surgeries, or endometriosis.
    - Treatment may involve surgery to repair the tubes or in vitro fertilization (IVF).

6. **Age-Related Infertility**
    - Fertility naturally declines with age, particularly after age 35.

- Options for older women include IVF, using donor eggs, and other assisted reproductive technologies.

For Men

1. **Low Sperm Count (Oligospermia)**
   - Low sperm count can be caused by various factors, including hormonal imbalances, genetic conditions, and lifestyle factors.
   - Treatment may involve lifestyle changes, medication, or assisted reproductive technologies like intracytoplasmic sperm injection (ICSI).
2. **Poor Sperm Motility (Asthenozoospermia)**
   - Poor sperm motility means that sperm have difficulty swimming to the egg.
   - Causes include lifestyle factors, infections, and genetic conditions.
   - Treatment may involve lifestyle changes, medication, or assisted reproductive technologies.
3. **Abnormal Sperm Morphology (Teratozoospermia)**
   - Abnormal sperm shape can affect the ability of sperm to fertilize the egg.
   - Causes include genetic factors, lifestyle factors, and environmental toxins.
   - Treatment may involve lifestyle changes, medication, or assisted reproductive technologies.

4. **Ejaculation Disorders**
   - Ejaculation disorders, such as premature ejaculation or retrograde ejaculation, can affect sperm delivery.
   - Treatment may involve medication, behavioral therapy, or assisted reproductive technologies.
5. **Varicocele**
   - Varicocele is an enlargement of veins within the scrotum that can affect sperm production.
   - Treatment options include surgery to repair the varicocele or assisted reproductive technologies.

For Both Partners

1. **Unexplained Infertility**
   - In some cases, no specific cause of infertility can be identified despite thorough evaluation.
   - Treatment options may include lifestyle changes, medication, or assisted reproductive technologies.
2. **Lifestyle Factors**
   - Lifestyle factors such as poor diet, lack of exercise, smoking, excessive alcohol consumption, and stress can affect fertility in both partners.
   - Addressing these factors can improve the chances of conception.
3. **Environmental Toxins**

- Exposure to environmental toxins, such as pesticides, heavy metals, and chemicals, can affect fertility in both partners.
- Reducing exposure to these toxins can improve reproductive health.

4. **Medical Conditions**
   - Chronic medical conditions, such as diabetes, thyroid disorders, and autoimmune diseases, can affect fertility in both partners.
   - Managing these conditions with the help of a healthcare provider can improve fertility.

Seeking Help for Fertility Challenges

If you have been trying to conceive for a year without success (or six months if you are over 35), it may be time to seek help from a fertility specialist. A fertility specialist can conduct a thorough evaluation to identify any underlying issues and recommend appropriate treatment options.

Treatment Options

1. **Medication**
   - Medications like clomiphene citrate and letrozole can stimulate ovulation in women with ovulation disorders.

- Hormonal treatments can address imbalances affecting fertility in both men and women.

2. **Surgery**
   - Surgical procedures can address structural issues affecting fertility, such as fibroids, endometriosis, and varicocele.

3. **Assisted Reproductive Technologies (ART)**
   - ART includes procedures like intrauterine insemination (IUI) and in vitro fertilization (IVF).
   - These technologies can help couples with various fertility challenges conceive.

4. **Lifestyle Changes**
   - Making positive lifestyle changes, such as improving diet, exercising regularly, and managing stress, can enhance fertility.

5. **Counseling and Support**
   - Infertility can be emotionally challenging. Seeking counseling and support from support groups or a mental health professional can help couples cope with the emotional aspects of infertility.

Fertility awareness is a crucial component of preparing for pregnancy. By understanding the menstrual cycle, tracking ovulation, enhancing fertility for both partners, and addressing common fertility challenges, couples can increase their chances of conceiving and having a healthy pregnancy. If fertility challenges arise, seeking help from a fertility specialist can provide the necessary support and treatment to achieve the dream of parenthood.

Chapter 4: Preparing Your Body for Pregnancy

Embarking on the journey to parenthood is a thrilling and transformative experience. Preparing your body for pregnancy is one of the most crucial steps in ensuring a healthy pregnancy and a healthy baby. This chapter will guide you through the essential aspects of getting your body ready, including the importance of folic acid and prenatal vitamins, maintaining a healthy weight, regular health checkups, oral health, and avoiding infections and illnesses.

Importance of Folic Acid and Prenatal Vitamins

Folic acid, a B vitamin, is critical for preventing neural tube defects, which are serious abnormalities of the brain and spine. The neural tube forms early in pregnancy, often before a woman even knows she is pregnant. Therefore, it is essential to start taking folic acid before conception.

Why Folic Acid?

Neural tube defects, such as spina bifida and anencephaly, occur very early in pregnancy, usually within the first month after conception. Folic acid helps form the neural tube properly, preventing these severe conditions. The Centers for Disease Control and Prevention (CDC) recommends that all women of reproductive age consume 400 micrograms (mcg) of folic acid daily. This can be achieved through a combination of diet and supplements.

Dietary Sources of Folic Acid

While folic acid supplements are essential, it is also beneficial to incorporate natural sources of folate (the natural form of folic acid) into your diet. Foods rich in folate include:

- Leafy green vegetables (spinach, kale, broccoli)
- Citrus fruits (oranges, lemons, grapefruits)
- Beans, peas, and lentils
- Fortified cereals and grains
- Nuts and seeds

Prenatal Vitamins

In addition to folic acid, prenatal vitamins are formulated to support the nutritional needs of a pregnant woman and her developing baby. They typically contain higher levels of certain nutrients than standard multivitamins. Key components of prenatal vitamins include:

- **Iron:** Vital for preventing anemia, which is common during pregnancy due to increased blood volume.

- **Calcium:** Essential for the development of strong bones and teeth in the baby, and to maintain the mother's bone health.
- **Vitamin D:** Supports bone health and immune function.
- **Iodine:** Important for brain development.
- **Omega-3 Fatty Acids:** Crucial for brain and eye development.

It is recommended to start taking prenatal vitamins at least three months before trying to conceive. This ensures that your body has an adequate supply of essential nutrients right from the start of pregnancy.

Maintaining a Healthy Weight

Your weight plays a significant role in your ability to conceive and maintain a healthy pregnancy. Both underweight and overweight conditions can pose risks to both mother and baby.

The Importance of a Healthy Weight

- **Underweight:** Women who are underweight may have irregular menstrual cycles, which can make it difficult to conceive. Additionally, being underweight can lead to insufficient nutrient stores for pregnancy, potentially affecting the baby's growth and development.

- **Overweight:** Women who are overweight or obese are at higher risk for several pregnancy complications, including gestational diabetes, high blood pressure, and preeclampsia. Excess weight can also affect fertility by causing hormonal imbalances that disrupt ovulation.

Calculating Your BMI

Body Mass Index (BMI) is a useful measure to determine if your weight is in a healthy range. You can calculate your BMI by dividing your weight in kilograms by your height in meters squared. A BMI between 18.5 and 24.9 is considered healthy.

Tips for Achieving and Maintaining a Healthy Weight

1. **Balanced Diet:** Focus on a diet rich in fruits, vegetables, whole grains, lean proteins, and healthy fats. Avoid highly processed foods, sugary beverages, and excessive intake of saturated and trans fats.
2. **Regular Exercise:** Aim for at least 150 minutes of moderate-intensity exercise per week. Activities like walking, swimming, and yoga are excellent choices.

3. **Consult a Nutritionist:** If you have specific dietary needs or challenges, a nutritionist can provide personalized guidance to help you achieve your weight goals.

Regular Health Checkups

Regular health checkups are a cornerstone of preconception care. They help identify and manage any health issues that could affect your pregnancy.

Pre-Pregnancy Checkup

Schedule a pre-pregnancy checkup with your healthcare provider. During this visit, your provider will review your medical history, current health status, and any medications you are taking. Key components of this checkup include:

- **Blood Tests:** To check for anemia, blood type, and infectious diseases.
- **Pap Smear and Pelvic Exam:** To screen for cervical abnormalities and assess the health of your reproductive organs.
- **Immunizations:** Ensure you are up-to-date on essential vaccines, such as the flu shot and MMR (measles, mumps, rubella).

Managing Chronic Conditions

If you have chronic health conditions like diabetes, hypertension, or thyroid disorders, it is crucial to manage these conditions before conceiving. Uncontrolled health issues can lead to complications during pregnancy. Work with your healthcare provider to develop a management plan that ensures your conditions are well-controlled.

Medication Review

Some medications are not safe to take during pregnancy. Discuss all prescription and over-the-counter medications with your healthcare provider. They can help you adjust your medication regimen to ensure it is safe for pregnancy.

Oral Health and Pregnancy

Oral health is often overlooked in preconception care, but it plays a vital role in overall health and pregnancy outcomes.

The Connection Between Oral Health and Pregnancy

Poor oral health can lead to infections that may affect pregnancy. For instance, periodontal disease (gum disease) has been linked to preterm birth and low birth weight. Additionally, hormonal changes during pregnancy can make gums more susceptible to inflammation and infection.

Preconception Dental Checkup

Visit your dentist for a preconception dental checkup. This allows your dentist to address any existing dental issues before you become pregnant. Key components of this checkup include:

- **Professional Cleaning:** To remove plaque and tartar buildup.
- **Examination:** To check for cavities, gum disease, and other dental problems.
- **X-Rays:** If needed, get dental X-rays done before pregnancy, as radiation exposure should be minimized during pregnancy.

Maintaining Oral Health During Pregnancy

- **Brushing and Flossing:** Brush your teeth twice daily with fluoride toothpaste and floss daily.
- **Healthy Diet:** Avoid sugary snacks and beverages that can contribute to tooth decay.
- **Regular Dental Visits:** Continue to see your dentist for routine checkups and cleanings during pregnancy.

Avoiding Infections and Illnesses

Preventing infections is crucial for a healthy pregnancy. Some infections can harm the developing baby or lead to complications.

Common Infections to Avoid

- **Rubella (German Measles):** Can cause serious birth defects if contracted during pregnancy. Ensure you are vaccinated before conceiving.
- **Chickenpox:** Another infection that can cause complications during pregnancy. Confirm your immunity with your healthcare provider.
- **Toxoplasmosis:** Caused by a parasite found in cat feces and undercooked meat. Avoid handling cat litter and ensure meat is cooked thoroughly.
- **Listeriosis:** A bacterial infection from contaminated food. Avoid unpasteurized dairy products, deli meats, and refrigerated smoked seafood.

Flu Vaccination

Getting the flu vaccine before or during pregnancy is essential. The flu can cause severe illness in pregnant women and lead to complications. The flu vaccine is safe during all trimesters of pregnancy.

COVID-19 Precautions

The COVID-19 pandemic has highlighted the importance of infection prevention. Follow public health guidelines to reduce your risk of contracting COVID-19. Discuss vaccination with your healthcare provider to ensure you are protected.

Good Hygiene Practices

- **Handwashing:** Wash your hands frequently with soap and water, especially after using the restroom, handling food, and being in public places.
- **Food Safety:** Wash fruits and vegetables thoroughly, cook meats to safe temperatures, and avoid cross-contamination in the kitchen.
- **Avoid Sick People:** Minimize contact with individuals who are sick, especially with contagious illnesses.

Managing Pre-Existing Infections

If you have chronic infections, such as HIV or hepatitis, work with your healthcare provider to manage these conditions before pregnancy. Proper management can reduce the risk of transmission to the baby and improve pregnancy outcomes.

Preparing your body for pregnancy is a multifaceted process that involves making healthy lifestyle choices, undergoing necessary medical checkups, and taking proactive steps to prevent infections. By prioritizing your health before conception, you can significantly enhance your chances of a healthy pregnancy and a healthy baby. This chapter has provided you with a comprehensive guide to the essential aspects of pre-pregnancy preparation. Remember, the journey to parenthood begins long before conception, and the efforts you make now will pave the way for a joyful and healthy pregnancy experience.

Chapter 6: Planning and Financial Preparation

Preparing for a baby involves more than just emotional and physical readiness; financial planning is also crucial. The costs associated with raising a child can be substantial, and planning ahead can help alleviate some of the financial stress that new parents often face. This chapter will guide you through budgeting for your baby, understanding insurance and medical costs, considering parental leave and work adjustments, and setting up a safe and comfortable home for your new arrival.

Budgeting for Baby

One of the first steps in financial preparation is creating a budget that accounts for the new expenses you'll incur once your baby arrives. This includes both one-time costs and ongoing expenses. Here's how to start:

1. **List One-Time Expenses**:
   - **Nursery Setup**: Crib, mattress, changing table, dresser, rocking chair, and decor.
   - **Baby Gear**: Stroller, car seat, baby carrier, high chair, and playpen.

- **Initial Clothing and Supplies**: Onesies, sleepwear, diapers, wipes, bottles, and formula if you plan to use it.
- **Health and Safety Items**: Baby monitor, first aid kit, and safety gates.
- **Maternity and Nursing Needs**: Maternity clothes, nursing bras, and breast pump.

2. **Calculate Ongoing Expenses**:
- **Diapers and Wipes**: Calculate how many you will need per month and their cost.
- **Formula and Baby Food**: If not breastfeeding, consider the cost of formula and later, baby food.
- **Childcare**: Daycare, nanny, or babysitting costs if both parents will be working.
- **Healthcare**: Regular pediatrician visits, vaccinations, and any potential medical emergencies.
- **Clothing and Supplies**: Babies grow quickly, so budget for new clothes and supplies as they age.
- **Miscellaneous**: Toys, books, and other educational materials.

3. **Establish a Savings Plan**:
- **Emergency Fund**: Ensure you have a robust emergency fund to cover unexpected expenses.

- **Long-Term Savings**: Start saving for future needs such as education and larger medical expenses.
- **Regular Contributions**: Set up automatic transfers to your savings account to ensure consistent contributions.

4. **Track Your Spending**:
   - **Monthly Review**: Regularly review your budget to ensure you are on track and adjust as necessary.
   - **Use Budgeting Tools**: Apps and spreadsheets can help you manage your expenses and stay organized.

Insurance and Medical Costs

Understanding your insurance and the potential medical costs associated with pregnancy and childbirth is essential. Here are key points to consider:

1. **Health Insurance**:
   - **Review Your Policy**: Understand what your health insurance covers, including prenatal care, labor and delivery, and postpartum care.
   - **Out-of-Pocket Costs**: Identify your deductibles, co-pays, and out-of-pocket maximums.

- **Add Baby to Your Policy**: Plan to add your baby to your health insurance policy as soon as they are born.

2. **Maternity and Delivery Costs**:
   - **Prenatal Care**: Routine visits, ultrasounds, and prenatal vitamins.
   - **Labor and Delivery**: Hospital stay, doctor's fees, anesthesia, and any potential complications.
   - **Postpartum Care**: Follow-up visits, lactation consulting, and any postpartum health issues.

3. **Pediatric Care**:
   - **Newborn Screenings**: Hearing tests, metabolic screenings, and immunizations.
   - **Regular Checkups**: Growth monitoring, developmental assessments, and routine vaccinations.

4. **Supplemental Insurance**:
   - **Disability Insurance**: Consider short-term disability insurance to cover income loss during maternity leave.
   - **Life Insurance**: Ensure both parents have adequate life insurance coverage to provide for the child in case of an untimely death.

5. **Flexible Spending Accounts (FSAs) and Health Savings Accounts (HSAs):**
   - **FSA**: Allows you to set aside pre-tax dollars for medical expenses not covered by insurance.
   - **HSA**: Available if you have a high-deductible health plan, offering tax advantages for medical expenses.

Parental Leave and Work Considerations

Balancing work and new parenting responsibilities is a critical aspect of planning for a baby. Here are the main considerations:

1. **Understanding Parental Leave Policies**:
   - **Employer Policies**: Check your employer's maternity and paternity leave policies, including the duration and whether it's paid or unpaid.
   - **State Laws**: Some states have specific laws that provide additional leave benefits beyond federal requirements.
2. **Family and Medical Leave Act (FMLA):**
   - **Eligibility**: FMLA provides up to 12 weeks of unpaid, job-protected leave for eligible employees.

- **Coverage**: Ensure you meet the eligibility requirements and understand how FMLA applies to your situation.

3. **Planning for Leave**:
   - **Timing**: Decide when to start your leave based on your due date and health.
   - **Communication**: Inform your employer about your leave plans well in advance to allow for necessary adjustments.
   - **Transition Plan**: Prepare a transition plan for your work responsibilities to ensure a smooth handover.

4. **Flexible Work Arrangements**:
   - **Remote Work**: Explore options for remote work or flexible hours to balance parenting and professional responsibilities.
   - **Part-Time Work**: Consider reducing your work hours temporarily if your job and financial situation allow it.
   - **Job Sharing**: Some employers may offer job-sharing arrangements where two employees share the responsibilities of one full-time position.

5. **Childcare Planning**:
   - **Daycare Centers**: Research and visit local daycare centers to find one that meets your needs and budget.

- **In-Home Care**: Consider hiring a nanny or babysitter for more personalized care.
- **Family Support**: If available, family members can provide reliable and cost-effective childcare.

Setting Up a Safe and Comfortable Home

Creating a safe and comfortable environment for your baby is crucial. This involves preparing the nursery, baby-proofing your home, and ensuring all essential items are in place.

1. **Preparing the Nursery**:
   - **Location**: Choose a room that is quiet and close to your bedroom.
   - **Furniture**: Invest in a sturdy crib, changing table, dresser, and a comfortable chair for feeding and rocking.
   - **Decor**: Keep it simple and soothing. Choose soft colors and avoid clutter.
2. **Baby-Proofing Your Home**:
   - **Safety Gates**: Install safety gates at the top and bottom of stairs.
   - **Electrical Outlets**: Cover all electrical outlets with safety plugs.
   - **Furniture Anchors**: Secure heavy furniture to the wall to prevent tipping.

- **Hazardous Substances**: Keep cleaning products, medications, and other hazardous substances out of reach.

3. **Essential Baby Items**:
   - **Clothing**: Stock up on onesies, sleepwear, socks, and hats. Choose soft, breathable fabrics.
   - **Diapering**: Have plenty of diapers, wipes, diaper cream, and a changing pad.
   - **Feeding**: Whether breastfeeding or formula feeding, have bottles, nipples, a breast pump, and a sterilizer.
   - **Bathing**: Get a baby bathtub, gentle baby soap, shampoo, and soft towels.
   - **Sleeping**: Ensure the crib mattress is firm and fits snugly. Avoid pillows, blankets, and stuffed animals in the crib.
4. **Health and Safety Items**:
   - **First Aid Kit**: Include baby-specific items like a digital thermometer, infant pain reliever, and nasal aspirator.
   - **Baby Monitor**: Choose a reliable baby monitor to keep an eye on your baby when you're not in the room.

- **Car Seat**: Ensure you have a car seat that meets safety standards and is properly installed.

5. **Comfort and Convenience**:
   - **Storage Solutions**: Organize baby clothes, toys, and supplies with bins, baskets, and shelves.
   - **Feeding Station**: Set up a designated area for feeding with a comfortable chair, a side table for supplies, and good lighting.
   - **Diapering Station**: Keep diapering supplies organized and within easy reach.

By taking these steps, you can ensure that your home is ready to welcome your new baby into a safe and comfortable environment. Proper planning and preparation will help you focus on enjoying the special moments with your newborn without unnecessary stress.

Financial and logistical planning for a new baby can seem overwhelming, but breaking it down into manageable steps can make the process more straightforward. By budgeting for baby expenses, understanding insurance and medical costs, planning for parental leave and work adjustments, and setting up a safe and comfortable home, you can create a stable and supportive environment for your growing family. This preparation will not only provide peace of mind but also allow you to focus on the joy and excitement of welcoming your new baby into the world.

Chapter 7: Mental and Emotional Preparation

Addressing Fears and Expectations

Embarking on the journey to parenthood is a significant life change that brings a mix of excitement, anticipation, and often, a fair share of fears and anxieties. It's completely normal to have concerns and expectations as you prepare for pregnancy and the arrival of your baby. Addressing these emotions early on can help you feel more in control and prepared for the changes ahead.

One of the most common fears is the uncertainty about the pregnancy itself. Many prospective parents worry about the health of their baby, the possibility of complications, and their own ability to handle the physical and emotional demands of pregnancy. It's important to acknowledge these fears rather than suppress them. Discussing them with your healthcare provider can provide reassurance and practical advice. Remember, regular prenatal care and following medical guidance significantly reduce the risks associated with pregnancy.

Another common concern is the fear of childbirth. The thought of labor and delivery can be daunting, especially if you're a first-time parent. Educating yourself about the process, understanding pain management options, and developing a birth plan can help alleviate some of this anxiety. Consider taking childbirth education classes, which offer detailed information about labor, delivery, and postpartum care. These classes also provide a platform to ask questions and voice your concerns.

Setting realistic expectations is crucial for your mental and emotional well-being. Pregnancy and parenthood often come with idealized images and societal pressures that can create unrealistic expectations. It's important to remember that every pregnancy is unique, and comparing yourself to others can lead to unnecessary stress.

Expectations around the physical changes during pregnancy can also be challenging. Your body will undergo significant transformations, and it's normal to feel self-conscious at times. Embrace these changes as part of the beautiful journey of bringing new life into the world. Surround yourself with supportive individuals who celebrate these changes with you.

Practicing mindfulness and relaxation techniques can be highly effective in managing fear and anxiety. Techniques such as deep breathing, meditation, and prenatal yoga can help calm your mind and body. These practices not only reduce stress but also prepare you for labor by enhancing your ability to focus and stay calm.

Journaling is another powerful tool to address your fears and expectations. Writing down your thoughts and feelings can provide clarity and a sense of relief. It allows you to process your emotions and track your journey, making it easier to see your growth and resilience over time.

If your fears and anxieties feel overwhelming, don't hesitate to seek professional support. Talking to a therapist who specializes in prenatal and postpartum care can be immensely beneficial. Therapy provides a safe space to explore your concerns, learn coping strategies, and receive emotional support.

Building a Support Network

A strong support network is vital for your mental and emotional well-being during pregnancy. Surrounding yourself with supportive individuals can make a significant difference in how you experience this transformative time.

Your support network can include a variety of people, such as your partner, family, friends, and healthcare providers. It's important to identify who you can rely on for different types of support. For instance, your partner may provide emotional and practical support, while your healthcare provider offers medical guidance and reassurance.

Family members, especially those who have experienced pregnancy, can be a great source of wisdom and comfort. Friends who are also parents can share their experiences and offer practical tips. It's helpful to have a mix of individuals who can provide emotional, informational, and tangible support.

Effective communication is key to building and maintaining a strong support network. Don't hesitate to express your needs and ask for help when necessary. Whether it's emotional support, assistance with household tasks, or just someone to listen, letting your support network know what you need can help you feel more supported and less isolated.

It's also important to set boundaries and communicate your preferences. Pregnancy can be a time when unsolicited advice is plentiful. Politely but firmly letting people know what kind of support and information you're looking for can help you maintain your emotional balance.

Joining a support group can provide additional layers of support and community. Support groups for expectant parents offer a space to share experiences, ask questions, and receive encouragement from others who are on the same journey. These groups can be found through local hospitals, community centers, or online platforms.

Online forums and social media groups dedicated to pregnancy and parenting can also be valuable resources. These communities often provide a wealth of information and a sense of camaraderie. However, it's important to approach online information with discernment and always cross-check with your healthcare provider.

Your healthcare providers play a crucial role in your support network. Regular check-ups and open communication with your doctor or midwife can provide reassurance and address any medical concerns you may have. Don't hesitate to ask questions and discuss your fears and expectations with them. They can provide evidence-based information and guide you through each stage of your pregnancy.

Building a support network also involves taking care of yourself. Self-care is not just about pampering yourself; it's about meeting your physical, emotional, and mental needs. Prioritize activities that bring you joy and relaxation, whether it's reading a book, taking a walk, or spending time with loved ones. Remember that taking care of yourself is essential for taking care of your baby.

Communicating with Your Partner

A strong, supportive partnership is one of the most significant assets during pregnancy. Open and honest communication with your partner can strengthen your relationship and help you both navigate the changes and challenges of pregnancy together.

It's important to share your fears and expectations with your partner. Open dialogue about what you're each experiencing can foster mutual understanding and support. Encourage your partner to share their thoughts and feelings as well. Remember that they may also have their own anxieties and expectations about pregnancy and parenthood.

Planning for your baby's arrival together can be a bonding experience. Discuss and make decisions about important topics such as childbirth plans, parenting styles, and how to divide responsibilities. Working together on these plans can help both of you feel more prepared and connected.

Pregnancy can bring physical and emotional changes that affect intimacy. It's important to maintain physical and emotional closeness during this time. Communicate openly about your needs and any discomforts you may be experiencing. Finding new ways to connect and support each other can help maintain intimacy and strengthen your relationship.

Support each other by being patient and understanding. Pregnancy can be a rollercoaster of emotions, and there will be times when you both need extra support. Small gestures of kindness and appreciation can go a long way in showing your partner that you care and are there for them.

Whenever possible, attend prenatal appointments together. This not only provides emotional support but also helps your partner stay informed and involved in the pregnancy journey. It's an opportunity for both of you to ask questions and receive guidance from your healthcare provider.

Discussing how you'll share parenting responsibilities is crucial. Talk about how you'll handle nighttime feedings, diaper changes, and other daily tasks. Having these conversations early can help set realistic expectations and prevent misunderstandings later on.

If you find that pregnancy is putting a strain on your relationship, consider seeking couple's counseling. A therapist can help you navigate the changes and challenges, improve communication, and strengthen your bond.

Preparing for Lifestyle Changes

Pregnancy and parenthood bring significant lifestyle changes. Preparing for these changes can help you adapt more smoothly and reduce stress.

Your daily routine will change as you prepare for the arrival of your baby. Consider how your schedule might shift to accommodate prenatal appointments, rest, and eventually, your baby's needs. Planning ahead can help you manage your time more effectively.

Preparing your home for your baby's arrival involves more than setting up a nursery. Consider safety measures such as baby-proofing your home, installing car seats, and ensuring a clean and comfortable environment. Having these preparations in place can help you feel more ready and less overwhelmed.

Pregnancy and raising a child come with financial considerations. Review your budget and start saving for expenses such as medical bills, baby supplies, and childcare. Financial planning can provide peace of mind and help you feel more secure as you prepare for parenthood.

Balancing work and family life is another important aspect of preparing for lifestyle changes. Consider discussing flexible work arrangements with your employer, such as adjusting your hours or working from home. This can help you manage your time better and reduce stress.

Physical and mental well-being are closely linked, and maintaining a healthy lifestyle is crucial during pregnancy. Continue to exercise regularly, eat a balanced diet, and get plenty of rest. These habits will not only benefit your physical health but also support your mental and emotional well-being.

Social support is an integral part of preparing for lifestyle changes. Lean on your support network for practical help and emotional support. Don't hesitate to ask for assistance with tasks such as household chores, errands, or babysitting. Sharing responsibilities can make the transition to parenthood smoother and less stressful.

Emotional preparation is just as important as practical preparation. Take time to reflect on the changes ahead and how you feel about them. It's normal to have a mix of emotions, including excitement, anxiety, and even fear. Acknowledging and addressing these feelings can help you feel more grounded and prepared.

Self-care is essential during this time. Make sure to take care of your own needs, whether it's through relaxation, hobbies, or spending time with loved ones. Remember that taking care of yourself is not selfish; it's necessary for your well-being and your ability to care for your baby.

Educate yourself about the changes and challenges of parenthood. Read books, attend parenting classes, and seek advice from experienced parents. The more informed you are, the more confident you'll feel as you navigate this new phase of life.

Finally, be patient with yourself and your partner. Adjusting to lifestyle changes takes time, and it's important to be compassionate and understanding with each other. Remember that it's okay to ask for help and to take things one step at a time.

By addressing fears and expectations, building a support network, communicating with your partner, and preparing for lifestyle changes, you can create a strong foundation for lifestyle changes, you can create a strong foundation for a healthy and confident pregnancy. This preparation will help you navigate the journey ahead with resilience and grace, ensuring a positive experience for both you and your baby.

Chapter 8: Pre-Pregnancy Health Checkups

Preparing for pregnancy involves taking several critical steps to ensure that both you and your future baby will be healthy. One of the most important steps in this process is undergoing thorough pre-pregnancy health checkups. These checkups can help identify and manage any potential health issues before they become problems during pregnancy. In this chapter, we will discuss the various components of pre-pregnancy health checkups, including physical exams and tests, blood tests and screening, pelvic exams and Pap smears, and reviewing medications and supplements.

Physical Exams and Tests

A comprehensive physical exam is a crucial part of pre-pregnancy health checkups. This exam helps your healthcare provider assess your overall health and identify any potential issues that could affect your pregnancy. During a physical exam, your healthcare provider will:

- **Assess Your General Health**: Your healthcare provider will review your medical history, including any chronic conditions, past surgeries, and previous pregnancies. They will also ask about your lifestyle, diet, exercise habits, and any use of tobacco, alcohol, or recreational drugs.

- **Measure Vital Signs**: Vital signs such as blood pressure, heart rate, respiratory rate, and temperature will be measured. High blood pressure, for example, can pose risks during pregnancy, so it's important to manage it beforehand.

- **Conduct a Physical Examination**: This includes checking your heart and lungs, examining your abdomen, and performing a breast exam. These checks can help detect any physical conditions that might need attention before pregnancy.

- **Evaluate Body Mass Index (BMI)**: Your weight and height will be measured to calculate your BMI. Maintaining a healthy weight is crucial for fertility and a healthy pregnancy. Your provider can offer guidance on achieving a healthy BMI through diet and exercise if necessary.

- **Review Vaccination Status**: Ensuring you are up-to-date on vaccinations is essential, as some vaccines cannot be given during pregnancy. Vaccines for rubella (German measles) and varicella (chickenpox) are particularly important, as contracting these diseases during pregnancy can lead to serious complications.

- **Discuss Lifestyle and Dietary Habits**: Your healthcare provider will talk to you about your lifestyle and dietary habits. They may recommend changes to ensure you are in the best possible health before conceiving.

- **Perform Additional Tests as Needed**: Depending on your health history and current health status, your provider may recommend additional tests such as an EKG (electrocardiogram) to check heart function, or a thyroid function test.

Blood Tests and Screening

Blood tests are a vital part of pre-pregnancy checkups, as they provide a wealth of information about your overall health and can detect potential issues that might affect pregnancy. Key blood tests and screenings include:

- **Complete Blood Count (CBC)**: This test measures various components of your blood, including red and white blood cells, hemoglobin, and platelets. It helps detect conditions like anemia, which can be managed before pregnancy to prevent complications.
- **Blood Type and Rh Factor**: Knowing your blood type and Rh factor is crucial. If you are Rh-negative and your partner is Rh-positive, there's a risk of Rh incompatibility, which can cause serious problems in future pregnancies. Your provider may recommend Rh immunoglobulin to prevent these issues.

- **Rubella Immunity**: This test checks for immunity to rubella. If you are not immune, you will need the rubella vaccine before getting pregnant, as rubella infection during pregnancy can lead to severe birth defects.

- **Hepatitis B and C Screening**: Screening for hepatitis B and C is important, as these infections can be transmitted to your baby during pregnancy or childbirth. If you have hepatitis, your provider will discuss ways to manage it during pregnancy.

- **Sexually Transmitted Infections (STIs)**: Testing for STIs such as HIV, syphilis, chlamydia, and gonorrhea is crucial, as untreated infections can cause complications during pregnancy and affect your baby's health. Early detection and treatment can prevent these issues.

- **Thyroid Function Tests**: Thyroid problems can affect fertility and pregnancy. Tests such as TSH (thyroid-stimulating hormone) and T4 (thyroxine) can detect hypo- or hyperthyroidism, allowing for appropriate treatment before pregnancy.

- **Diabetes Screening**: If you have risk factors for diabetes, such as a family history or being overweight, your provider may recommend a fasting blood glucose test or HbA1c test to check for diabetes or prediabetes. Managing blood sugar levels before pregnancy is crucial for preventing complications.

- **Genetic Carrier Screening**: Depending on your family history and ethnicity, your provider may recommend genetic screening for conditions such as cystic fibrosis, sickle cell anemia, or Tay-Sachs disease. Identifying genetic risks allows for informed decision-making and planning.

Pelvic Exams and Pap Smears

Pelvic exams and Pap smears are essential components of pre-pregnancy health checkups. These tests help ensure that your reproductive organs are healthy and identify any issues that need to be addressed before conception.

- **Pelvic Exam**: During a pelvic exam, your healthcare provider will check your external and internal reproductive organs, including the vulva, vagina, cervix, uterus, and ovaries. This exam helps detect conditions such as fibroids, ovarian cysts, or infections that could affect your ability to conceive or maintain a healthy pregnancy.
- **Pap Smear**: A Pap smear (or Pap test) is a procedure to collect cells from your cervix, the lower part of your uterus that opens into the vagina. The cells are examined under a microscope to check for abnormalities that could indicate cervical cancer or

pre-cancerous changes. It's important to address any abnormal results before becoming pregnant, as treatments during pregnancy can be more complicated.

- **Human Papillomavirus (HPV) Test**: Often performed alongside a Pap smear, this test checks for the presence of HPV, a virus that can cause cervical cancer. If HPV is detected, your provider will discuss further testing or monitoring.
- **Screening for Infections**: Your provider may test for infections that could affect your reproductive health, such as bacterial vaginosis, yeast infections, or sexually transmitted infections (STIs). Treating these infections before pregnancy reduces the risk of complications.
- **Assessment of the Uterus and Ovaries**: During the pelvic exam, your provider will check for any abnormalities in the size or shape of your uterus and ovaries. Conditions such as uterine fibroids or ovarian cysts can affect fertility and pregnancy. If any abnormalities are found, your provider may recommend further evaluation or treatment.

Reviewing Medications and Supplements

Reviewing your current medications and supplements is a critical step in pre-pregnancy planning. Certain medications and supplements can affect fertility or pose risks during pregnancy, so it's essential to ensure that everything you are taking is safe.

- **Prescription Medications**: Inform your healthcare provider about all prescription medications you are currently taking. Some medications may need to be adjusted or discontinued before pregnancy, while others may be perfectly safe. For example, certain blood pressure medications, acne treatments, and anti-seizure medications can be harmful during pregnancy and may need to be replaced with safer alternatives.

- **Over-the-Counter Medications**: Over-the-counter medications, including pain relievers, cold remedies, and allergy medications, should also be reviewed. Some may not be safe during pregnancy or may need to be taken in lower doses. Your provider can recommend safe alternatives if necessary.

- **Supplements and Herbal Products**: Many people take supplements and herbal products for various health reasons. However, not all supplements are safe during pregnancy. For example, high doses of vitamin A can be harmful, and some herbal products can affect hormone levels or cause uterine contractions. It's important to discuss all supplements with your provider to ensure they are safe to continue.

- **Prenatal Vitamins**: Starting a prenatal vitamin before conception is recommended to ensure you are getting essential nutrients for a healthy pregnancy. Prenatal vitamins typically contain folic acid, iron, calcium, and other important nutrients. Folic acid is especially crucial, as it helps prevent neural tube defects in the developing baby.

- **Medications for Chronic Conditions**: If you have a chronic condition such as diabetes, epilepsy, or high blood pressure, managing these conditions effectively before pregnancy is crucial. Your provider will work with you to adjust medications and develop a management plan that ensures your health and the health of your baby during pregnancy.

- **Immunizations**: Review your immunization status with your provider. Vaccines such as the flu vaccine and Tdap (tetanus, diphtheria, and pertussis) are safe and recommended during pregnancy. However, some vaccines, like the rubella and varicella vaccines, should be administered before conception.

Preparing for pregnancy involves taking proactive steps to ensure that you are in the best possible health before conceiving. Pre-pregnancy health checkups play a vital role in this preparation by identifying and managing any potential health issues that could affect your pregnancy. By undergoing physical exams and tests, blood tests and screenings, pelvic exams and Pap smears, and reviewing medications and supplements, you can create a healthy foundation for a successful pregnancy. Working closely with your healthcare provider and making necessary lifestyle changes can help you embark on your pregnancy journey with confidence and peace of mind.

Chapter 9: Lifestyle Adjustments for a Healthy Pregnancy

Quitting Smoking, Alcohol, and Drugs

Smoking

Smoking during pregnancy is highly detrimental to both maternal and fetal health. Tobacco smoke contains thousands of chemicals, including nicotine, carbon monoxide, and tar, all of which can cross the placenta and affect the developing baby. Smoking increases the risk of miscarriage, preterm birth, low birth weight, stillbirth, and sudden infant death syndrome (SIDS). Moreover, smoking can lead to complications such as placental abruption, where the placenta detaches from the uterus wall prematurely, causing severe bleeding.

Quitting smoking is challenging, but it's one of the most critical steps a pregnant woman can take for her health and the health of her baby. Here are some strategies to help quit smoking:

1. **Seek Professional Help**: Consulting with a healthcare provider can provide access to resources such as counseling, support groups, and medications that can assist in quitting smoking.

2. **Behavioral Therapy**: Cognitive-behavioral therapy (CBT) can help address the psychological aspects of nicotine addiction by changing thought patterns and behaviors related to smoking.
3. **Nicotine Replacement Therapy (NRT)**: While pregnant women should avoid nicotine, NRT can be considered if smoking cessation proves particularly difficult. It's crucial to use NRT under medical supervision.
4. **Support Systems**: Engaging family, friends, and support groups can provide encouragement and accountability.
5. **Avoid Triggers**: Identifying and avoiding situations that trigger the urge to smoke, such as social gatherings with smokers or stressful situations, can be beneficial.

Alcohol

Alcohol consumption during pregnancy can lead to severe developmental problems in the fetus. The most severe consequence is fetal alcohol spectrum disorders (FASD), which include physical, behavioral, and learning disabilities. Alcohol can interfere with the development of the baby's brain and other critical organs, leading to lifelong challenges.

To ensure a healthy pregnancy, it is advised to abstain from alcohol entirely. Here are some tips for quitting alcohol:

1. **Understand the Risks**: Educating yourself about the effects of alcohol on fetal development can reinforce the importance of abstinence.
2. **Seek Support**: Joining support groups such as Alcoholics Anonymous (AA) or seeking counseling can provide the necessary support to quit alcohol.
3. **Substitute with Healthy Alternatives**: Replace alcoholic beverages with non-alcoholic options such as sparkling water, herbal teas, or non-alcoholic cocktails.
4. **Avoid Tempting Situations**: Steering clear of environments where alcohol is present can help reduce temptation.
5. **Professional Help**: If quitting alcohol is challenging, seek help from a healthcare provider who can offer resources and support.

Recreational Drugs

The use of recreational drugs during pregnancy poses significant risks to both the mother and the baby. Drugs such as marijuana, cocaine, heroin, and methamphetamine can lead to a variety of complications, including preterm birth, low birth weight, developmental delays, and withdrawal symptoms in newborns.

To ensure a drug-free pregnancy, consider the following steps:

1. **Seek Medical Advice**: Consult a healthcare provider for guidance and support in quitting drug use. They can refer you to appropriate treatment programs and resources.
2. **Therapy and Counseling**: Behavioral therapies and counseling can help address the underlying issues contributing to drug use and provide strategies for quitting.
3. **Support Groups**: Joining support groups for individuals struggling with substance abuse can provide a sense of community and encouragement.
4. **Rehabilitation Programs**: In severe cases, enrolling in a rehabilitation program can offer comprehensive support and treatment to quit drug use.
5. **Avoid Triggers and High-Risk Situations**: Identifying and avoiding situations or people associated with drug use can help reduce the risk of relapse.

Reducing Caffeine Intake

Caffeine is a stimulant found in coffee, tea, chocolate, and many soft drinks and energy drinks. While moderate caffeine consumption is generally considered safe, excessive intake during pregnancy has been linked to an increased risk of miscarriage, preterm birth, low birth weight, and developmental issues.

The American College of Obstetricians and Gynecologists (ACOG) recommends limiting caffeine intake to no more than 200 milligrams per day during pregnancy, which is approximately the amount found in one 12-ounce cup of coffee. Here are some strategies to reduce caffeine intake:

1. **Switch to Decaffeinated Options**: Choose decaffeinated coffee, tea, and other beverages to satisfy your cravings without the high caffeine content.
2. **Monitor Caffeine Sources**: Be mindful of hidden sources of caffeine such as chocolate, certain medications, and soft drinks. Reading labels can help you track your total caffeine intake.
3. **Gradual Reduction**: If you are used to consuming large amounts of caffeine, reduce your intake gradually to avoid withdrawal symptoms such as headaches and irritability.
4. **Healthy Alternatives**: Substitute caffeinated drinks with herbal teas, water, or milk to ensure adequate hydration and nutrition.
5. **Stay Hydrated**: Drinking plenty of water can help reduce the desire for caffeinated beverages and keep you hydrated.

Safe Foods

Maintaining a healthy diet during pregnancy is crucial for the development of the baby and the well-being of the mother. Here are some safe food choices that provide essential nutrients:

1. **Fruits and Vegetables**: Rich in vitamins, minerals, and fiber. Aim for a variety of colors to ensure a wide range of nutrients.
2. **Whole Grains**: Foods such as oatmeal, brown rice, and whole wheat bread provide energy and fiber.
3. **Lean Proteins**: Sources include poultry, lean beef, tofu, beans, and legumes. These are important for the baby's growth and development.
4. **Dairy Products**: Milk, cheese, and yogurt provide calcium and vitamin D, essential for bone health.
5. **Healthy Fats**: Include sources like avocados, nuts, seeds, and olive oil for essential fatty acids.

Unsafe Foods

Certain foods should be avoided during pregnancy due to the risk of contamination or harmful effects on the baby. Here are some foods to steer clear of:

1. **Raw or Undercooked Meat and Eggs**: These can harbor harmful bacteria such as Salmonella and E. coli. Ensure all meats are cooked thoroughly, and eggs are fully cooked.
2. **Unpasteurized Dairy Products**: These can contain Listeria, which can cause miscarriage or severe illness in newborns. Always choose pasteurized products.
3. **Certain Fish**: Avoid high-mercury fish such as shark, swordfish, king mackerel, and tilefish. Instead, opt for low-mercury fish like salmon, sardines, and trout.
4. **Deli Meats and Hot Dogs**: These can also harbor Listeria. If consumed, they should be heated until steaming hot.
5. **Raw Sprouts**: Alfalfa, clover, and radish sprouts can be contaminated with bacteria. It's best to avoid them unless fully cooked.
6. **Caffeine and Alcohol**: As previously discussed, limit caffeine and avoid alcohol entirely.

Environmental Factors to Avoid

Chemical Exposures

Pregnant women should avoid exposure to certain chemicals that can harm the developing baby. These include:

1. **Pesticides and Herbicides**: These chemicals can be harmful if inhaled or absorbed through the skin. Avoid using them in your home and garden.
2. **Household Cleaners**: Some cleaning products contain harsh chemicals. Opt for natural or homemade cleaning solutions.
3. **Paint Fumes**: Exposure to paint fumes, especially from oil-based paints and solvents, can be harmful. If painting is necessary, ensure the area is well-ventilated, or consider hiring someone to do it.
4. **Personal Care Products**: Some cosmetics and personal care products contain harmful chemicals. Choose products that are labeled as safe for pregnancy.

Radiation and Heat

Exposure to high levels of radiation and excessive heat can pose risks during pregnancy. Consider the following precautions:

1. **X-Rays**: If an X-ray is necessary, inform the technician of your pregnancy so they can take appropriate precautions.
2. **Hot Tubs and Saunas**: Prolonged exposure to high temperatures can increase the risk of neural tube defects. It's best to avoid hot tubs and saunas during pregnancy.

3. **Electronic Devices**: While everyday use of electronic devices is generally considered safe, it's wise to avoid prolonged exposure to electromagnetic fields from high-power sources.

Infectious Agents

Pregnant women should take precautions to avoid infections that can affect the baby. Key steps include:

1. **Hand Hygiene**: Wash hands frequently, especially after handling raw meat, using the bathroom, or caring for sick individuals.
2. **Vaccinations**: Ensure vaccinations are up to date before pregnancy. Avoid live vaccines during pregnancy and consult your healthcare provider about which vaccines are safe.
3. **Animal Contact**: Avoid handling cat litter, which can contain Toxoplasma gondii, a parasite that can cause toxoplasmosis. Also, avoid contact with sick animals.

Workplace Hazards

If you work in an environment with potential hazards, take the following precautions:

1. **Chemical Exposure**: If your job involves exposure to chemicals, ensure proper safety measures are in place and discuss any concerns with your employer.
2. **Physical Strain**: Avoid heavy lifting, prolonged standing, or repetitive strenuous activities that can cause strain or injury.
3. **Radiation**: If you work in a healthcare setting or another environment with potential radiation exposure, follow all safety protocols to minimize risk.

Travel Considerations

Traveling during pregnancy can be safe, but certain precautions should be taken:

1. **Vaccinations and Health Risks**: If traveling abroad, check for any required vaccinations and potential health risks. Avoid travel to areas with Zika virus or other significant health concerns.
2. **Travel Insurance**: Consider purchasing travel insurance that covers pregnancy-related issues.
3. **Comfort and Safety**: During travel, stay hydrated, take frequent breaks to move around, and wear seat belts properly.

In summary, making lifestyle adjustments for a healthy pregnancy involves quitting smoking, alcohol, and drugs;

reducing caffeine intake; consuming safe foods; and avoiding harmful environmental factors. By adopting these practices, you can create a healthy environment for your baby's development and ensure a smoother pregnancy journey. Always consult with your healthcare provider for personalized advice and support tailored to your specific needs.

Chapter 10: Special Considerations

Pre-existing Medical Conditions

When planning for pregnancy, it is crucial to consider any pre-existing medical conditions that may affect your health or the health of your baby. Pre-existing conditions can complicate pregnancy, but with proper management and care, many women with chronic health issues can still have a healthy pregnancy and baby.

Diabetes Women with diabetes need to ensure their blood sugar levels are well-controlled before conceiving. Poorly controlled diabetes can increase the risk of birth defects, miscarriage, preterm birth, and other complications. It is essential to work closely with your healthcare provider to monitor your blood sugar levels, adjust medications if necessary, and follow a healthy diet and exercise plan. Regular checkups and prenatal visits will help manage your diabetes throughout the pregnancy.

Hypertension (High Blood Pressure) High blood pressure can pose risks such as preeclampsia, preterm delivery, and placental abruption. If you have hypertension, it is important to manage your blood pressure through lifestyle changes and medications if prescribed. Your healthcare provider may recommend more frequent prenatal visits to monitor your blood pressure and the baby's development.

Maintaining a low-sodium diet, regular physical activity, and stress management techniques can also help control blood pressure levels.

Epilepsy Epilepsy and the medications used to control seizures can affect pregnancy. Certain antiepileptic drugs may increase the risk of birth defects, so it is vital to discuss your medication regimen with your healthcare provider before conceiving. Your doctor may adjust your medications to find the safest options for both you and your baby. Regular monitoring and a detailed birth plan can help manage epilepsy during pregnancy.

Asthma Asthma symptoms can worsen during pregnancy, affecting both the mother and the baby. It is important to continue using prescribed asthma medications and to work with your healthcare provider to manage your condition. Avoiding asthma triggers, following a healthy lifestyle, and attending regular prenatal checkups can help keep asthma under control.

Thyroid Disorders Both hypothyroidism (underactive thyroid) and hyperthyroidism (overactive thyroid) can affect pregnancy. Thyroid hormones are crucial for fetal development, especially brain development. Women with thyroid disorders need to have their thyroid function closely monitored and medications adjusted as necessary.

Regular blood tests and prenatal visits will help ensure optimal thyroid hormone levels throughout the pregnancy.

Autoimmune Diseases Autoimmune diseases such as lupus, rheumatoid arthritis, and multiple sclerosis can pose challenges during pregnancy. The symptoms of these conditions may flare up or improve during pregnancy. It is essential to work with a healthcare provider who specializes in high-risk pregnancies to manage these conditions. Medications may need to be adjusted, and close monitoring will help address any complications that arise.

Mental Health Conditions Mental health conditions, including depression, anxiety, and bipolar disorder, can impact pregnancy and postpartum well-being. It is important to discuss your mental health history with your healthcare provider and continue any prescribed treatments. Mental health support, counseling, and a strong support system can help manage these conditions during pregnancy and beyond.

Obesity Obesity increases the risk of complications such as gestational diabetes, preeclampsia, and cesarean delivery. Women with a high BMI should aim to achieve a healthy weight before conceiving. A balanced diet, regular exercise, and working with a healthcare provider can help manage weight during pregnancy. Regular prenatal visits will monitor the health of both the mother and the baby.

Heart Disease Pregnancy places additional strain on the heart, which can be challenging for women with pre-existing heart conditions. It is crucial to consult a cardiologist before conceiving to assess your heart health and develop a management plan. Close monitoring throughout pregnancy will help manage the risks and ensure the health of both mother and baby.

High-Risk Pregnancy Factors

A high-risk pregnancy is one that poses increased health risks to the mother or baby. Various factors can contribute to a high-risk pregnancy, and understanding these risks can help you take steps to mitigate them.

Advanced Maternal Age Women aged 35 and older are considered to have a higher risk of pregnancy complications, including chromosomal abnormalities, gestational diabetes, preeclampsia, and preterm birth. Advanced maternal age also increases the likelihood of needing a cesarean delivery. Regular prenatal care, early and consistent monitoring, and specialized screenings can help manage these risks.

Multiple Pregnancies Carrying more than one baby (twins, triplets, or higher-order multiples) significantly increases the risk of complications such as preterm birth, low birth weight, gestational diabetes, and preeclampsia.

Women with multiple pregnancies require more frequent prenatal visits and specialized care to monitor the health and development of each baby. Bed rest or reduced physical activity may be recommended to reduce the risk of preterm labor.

History of Pregnancy Complications Women who have experienced previous pregnancy complications, such as preterm birth, stillbirth, or preeclampsia, are at a higher risk of similar issues in subsequent pregnancies. It is important to inform your healthcare provider about your pregnancy history so that they can closely monitor your health and take preventive measures. Early and regular prenatal care, along with personalized management plans, can help reduce the risk of recurrence.

Chronic Health Conditions Pre-existing medical conditions, as discussed earlier, can make a pregnancy high-risk. Women with conditions such as diabetes, hypertension, kidney disease, or autoimmune disorders require specialized care and close monitoring throughout pregnancy. Managing these conditions effectively can help ensure a healthier pregnancy and reduce complications.

Lifestyle Factors Certain lifestyle factors, such as smoking, alcohol consumption, and drug use, can significantly increase the risk of pregnancy complications. Quitting smoking, avoiding alcohol and recreational drugs, and adopting a healthy lifestyle before and during pregnancy can help mitigate these risks.

Obesity Obesity is a major risk factor for high-risk pregnancies. Women with obesity are more likely to develop gestational diabetes, preeclampsia, and have larger babies, which can complicate delivery. Achieving a healthy weight before pregnancy and maintaining it through a balanced diet and regular exercise can help reduce these risks.

Infections Infections such as sexually transmitted infections (STIs), urinary tract infections, and certain viral infections (e.g., Zika virus, COVID-19) can pose significant risks during pregnancy. Early detection and treatment of infections, along with preventive measures such as vaccinations and avoiding exposure, can help protect both the mother and the baby.

Blood Clotting Disorders Conditions such as thrombophilia or antiphospholipid syndrome increase the risk of blood clots during pregnancy, which can lead to complications such as preeclampsia, fetal growth restriction, or miscarriage. Women with blood clotting disorders require specialized care and may need to take blood-thinning medications during pregnancy.

Abnormal Placenta Placenta previa (where the placenta covers the cervix) and placental abruption (where the placenta detaches from the uterine wall) are serious conditions that can cause bleeding and pose risks to both the mother and baby. Women with abnormal placental conditions need close monitoring and may require bed rest or early delivery to ensure safety.

Fetal Health Issues Conditions such as fetal growth restriction, congenital abnormalities, or genetic disorders can classify a pregnancy as high-risk. Specialized prenatal care, including advanced imaging and genetic testing, can help monitor and manage these conditions to optimize outcomes for the baby.

Multiple Pregnancies

Multiple pregnancies, such as twins, triplets, or higher-order multiples, come with unique challenges and increased risks. Understanding these challenges and working closely with your healthcare provider can help ensure a healthy pregnancy and delivery.

Increased Risk of Preterm Birth One of the most significant risks associated with multiple pregnancies is preterm birth. Multiple pregnancies are more likely to result in premature delivery, which can lead to complications for the babies, such as respiratory distress syndrome, developmental delays, and other health issues. Women carrying multiples should be prepared for the possibility of preterm labor and may need to take preventive measures, such as bed rest or reduced physical activity.

Low Birth Weight Babies born from multiple pregnancies are often smaller and have a lower birth weight than singletons. Low birth weight can increase the risk of health problems and require specialized care after birth. Regular prenatal visits and ultrasounds can help monitor the growth and development of each baby.

Gestational Diabetes Women with multiple pregnancies have a higher risk of developing gestational diabetes. Gestational diabetes can lead to larger babies, increasing the risk of delivery complications. Managing blood sugar levels through diet, exercise, and medication if necessary is crucial for women with multiple pregnancies.

Preeclampsia The risk of preeclampsia, a condition characterized by high blood pressure and organ damage, is higher in multiple pregnancies. Preeclampsia can lead to serious complications for both the mother and babies if not managed properly. Regular monitoring of blood pressure and other symptoms is essential.

Fetal Growth Restriction Fetal growth restriction, where one or more babies do not grow at the expected rate, is more common in multiple pregnancies. This condition requires close monitoring through ultrasounds and may necessitate early delivery if the babies are not growing adequately.

Delivery Considerations Women with multiple pregnancies are more likely to require a cesarean delivery due to the increased risk of complications during vaginal birth. It is important to discuss delivery options and create a birth plan with your healthcare provider. In some cases, a combination of vaginal and cesarean delivery may be necessary, depending on the position and health of the babies.

Emotional and Physical Support Carrying multiples can be physically demanding and emotionally challenging. It is important to have a strong support system in place, including family, friends, and healthcare professionals. Seeking support from multiple pregnancy support groups can also provide valuable information and emotional support.

Nutritional Needs Women with multiple pregnancies have higher nutritional needs to support the growth and development of each baby. It is important to follow a well-balanced diet rich in essential nutrients, including folic acid, iron, calcium, and protein. Your healthcare provider may recommend additional supplements to meet these increased nutritional demands.

Age-Related Considerations

The age of the mother can significantly impact pregnancy and childbirth. Women of different age groups face unique challenges and considerations when planning for pregnancy.

Teen Pregnancy Teen pregnancy, defined as pregnancy in women aged 19 and younger, is associated with higher risks of complications such as preterm birth, low birth weight, and preeclampsia. Teenage mothers are also more likely to experience socioeconomic challenges, including limited access to healthcare, education, and financial stability. It is important for teenage mothers to receive comprehensive prenatal care, education, and support to address these challenges and ensure a healthy pregnancy and baby.

Women Aged 20-34 This age group is generally considered the optimal reproductive age, with lower risks of pregnancy complications compared to younger and older age groups. However, maintaining a healthy lifestyle, regular prenatal care, and addressing any pre-existing medical conditions remain important for all women, regardless of age.

Women Aged 35 and Older Women aged 35 and older are considered to have advanced maternal age, which is associated with increased risks of complications such as chromosomal abnormalities (e.g., Down syndrome), gestational diabetes, preeclampsia, and preterm birth. Advanced maternal age also increases the likelihood of requiring fertility treatments to conceive. Regular prenatal care, specialized screenings, and close monitoring can help manage these risks and ensure a healthy pregnancy.

Women Aged 40 and Older Pregnancy after the age of 40 comes with additional challenges, including a higher risk of infertility, miscarriage, chromosomal abnormalities, and pregnancy complications such as high blood pressure and gestational diabetes. Women in this age group may require fertility treatments such as in vitro fertilization (IVF) to conceive. Comprehensive prenatal care, including advanced screenings and regular monitoring, is essential to manage these risks and support a healthy pregnancy.

Considerations for Older Fathers While the age of the mother is often the primary focus, the age of the father can also impact pregnancy outcomes. Advanced paternal age, typically defined as 40 years and older, is associated with an increased risk of genetic mutations, autism spectrum disorders, and certain psychiatric conditions in offspring. It is important for older fathers to be aware of these risks and discuss them with their healthcare provider.

Pregnancy is a complex journey that requires careful planning and consideration of various factors to ensure the health and well-being of both the mother and baby. Special considerations such as pre-existing medical conditions, high-risk pregnancy factors, multiple pregnancies, and age-related challenges require additional attention and care.

By working closely with healthcare providers, maintaining a healthy lifestyle, and being proactive in managing risks, expectant parents can navigate these challenges and enjoy a healthy and confident pregnancy journey. Remember, every pregnancy is unique, and individualized care and support are essential to achieving the best possible outcomes for you and your baby.

When to Stop Birth Control

Deciding when to stop birth control is an important step in the journey to conception. The timing can vary based on the type of contraceptive method used and individual health considerations. It's essential to understand how different birth control methods affect your body and fertility.

Hormonal Birth Control Hormonal contraceptives, such as the pill, patch, ring, implant, and certain intrauterine devices (IUDs), can influence your menstrual cycle. These methods work by regulating hormones to prevent ovulation. When you stop using hormonal birth control, your body may need time to readjust and return to its natural cycle.

- **Birth Control Pills**: It's typically recommended to stop taking birth control pills a few months before you plan to conceive. This period allows your menstrual cycle to normalize and helps in tracking ovulation. While some women may resume regular cycles immediately, others might take a few months.
- **Birth Control Patch and Ring**: Similar to the pill, it's advisable to stop using the patch or ring a few months before trying to conceive to allow your hormones to regulate.

- **Birth Control Implant**: The implant can be removed at any time, but it may take a few weeks to a few months for ovulation to return.
- **Hormonal IUD**: After removing a hormonal IUD, some women might begin ovulating within a month, while for others, it might take longer.

Non-Hormonal Birth Control Non-hormonal methods, such as the copper IUD (Paragard), barrier methods (condoms, diaphragms), and natural family planning, typically do not affect hormone levels. Fertility usually returns immediately after stopping these methods.

- **Copper IUD**: Fertility can return almost immediately after removal.
- **Barrier Methods**: These methods do not interfere with hormones, so there's no delay in fertility once they are discontinued.

Considerations for Stopping Birth Control It's crucial to consult with your healthcare provider before stopping birth control. They can provide personalized advice based on your health history and the type of contraceptive you've been using. Additionally, they can help you understand what to expect and how to monitor your menstrual cycle and ovulation post-contraception.

Timing intercourse to align with ovulation increases the chances of conception. Understanding your menstrual cycle and identifying your fertile window are key components in achieving pregnancy.

Understanding the Menstrual Cycle A typical menstrual cycle lasts between 21 and 35 days, with the average being around 28 days. The cycle begins on the first day of menstruation and ends the day before the next period starts. Ovulation, the release of an egg from the ovary, typically occurs around the midpoint of the cycle.

Identifying the Fertile Window The fertile window is the period during which conception is most likely to occur. This window usually spans six days: five days before ovulation and the day of ovulation. Sperm can survive in the female reproductive tract for up to five days, while the egg is viable for about 12-24 hours after ovulation.

Methods to Track Ovulation There are several methods to identify ovulation and determine the fertile window:

- **Calendar Method**: Track your menstrual cycle over several months to predict ovulation. Ovulation usually occurs about 14 days before the next period.

For example, in a 28-day cycle, ovulation would likely occur around day 14.

- **Basal Body Temperature (BBT)**: Measure your body temperature every morning before getting out of bed. A slight increase in BBT, typically around 0.5 to 1 degree Fahrenheit, indicates ovulation has occurred.
- **Cervical Mucus**: Observe changes in cervical mucus. Around ovulation, cervical mucus becomes clear, stretchy, and similar to egg whites, indicating peak fertility.
- **Ovulation Predictor Kits (OPKs)**: These kits detect the surge in luteinizing hormone (LH) that precedes ovulation. A positive result suggests that ovulation will occur within the next 12-36 hours.

Optimal Timing for Intercourse For the best chance of conception, aim to have intercourse during the fertile window. Ideally, have sex every other day starting a few days before the expected ovulation and continuing until a few days after. Regular intercourse during this period maximizes the likelihood of sperm meeting the egg.

Dealing with Infertility

Infertility can be a challenging and emotional experience for couples trying to conceive. It's defined as the inability to achieve pregnancy after one year of regular, unprotected intercourse for women under 35, and after six months for women 35 and older. Understanding the causes and seeking appropriate help is crucial in managing infertility.

Common Causes of Infertility Infertility can result from factors affecting either partner or both. Common causes include:

- **Female Factors**:
  - **Ovulatory Disorders**: Conditions such as polycystic ovary syndrome (PCOS), thyroid disorders, and premature ovarian failure can disrupt ovulation.
  - **Tubal Blockages**: Blocked fallopian tubes can prevent the egg and sperm from meeting. This can be due to infections, endometriosis, or pelvic inflammatory disease (PID).
  - **Uterine or Cervical Issues**: Fibroids, polyps, or abnormalities in the uterus or cervix can hinder implantation or sperm passage.
  - **Age**: As women age, the quantity and quality of eggs decrease, reducing fertility.
- **Male Factors**:
  - **Sperm Disorders**: Low sperm count, poor motility, or abnormal morphology can affect fertility.

- **Ejaculation Issues**: Conditions such as retrograde ejaculation or blockage of the ejaculatory ducts can prevent sperm from being expelled.
- **Hormonal Imbalances**: Hormones such as testosterone, FSH, and LH play crucial roles in sperm production and function.

Diagnosis and Testing If you suspect infertility, it's essential to seek medical evaluation. Diagnostic tests can identify underlying issues and guide treatment. Common tests include:

- **Female Testing**:
  - **Ovulation Testing**: Blood tests to measure hormone levels, such as LH, FSH, and progesterone, can confirm ovulation.
  - **Hysterosalpingography (HSG)**: An X-ray procedure that checks for blockages in the fallopian tubes.
  - **Ultrasound**: Imaging to assess the uterus, ovaries, and follicles.
  - **Laparoscopy**: A surgical procedure to examine the pelvic organs and detect conditions like endometriosis.
- **Male Testing**:
  - **Semen Analysis**: Evaluates sperm count, motility, morphology, and volume.

- **Hormonal Testing**: Blood tests to assess hormone levels affecting sperm production.
- **Genetic Testing**: Identifies genetic causes of infertility.

Treatment Options Treatment for infertility depends on the underlying cause and may involve lifestyle changes, medication, surgery, or assisted reproductive technologies (ART).

- **Lifestyle Changes**: Improving diet, exercise, and reducing stress can enhance fertility. Avoiding smoking, alcohol, and recreational drugs is also crucial.
- **Medications**: Fertility drugs, such as Clomiphene (Clomid) or Letrozole, can stimulate ovulation. Gonadotropins may be prescribed for more complex issues.
- **Surgery**: Surgical procedures can correct anatomical issues, such as removing fibroids or treating endometriosis.
- **Assisted Reproductive Technologies (ART)**: In cases where other treatments are ineffective, ART methods like intrauterine insemination (IUI) or in vitro fertilization (IVF) can be used.

Assisted Reproductive Technologies

Assisted Reproductive Technologies (ART) encompass a range of medical procedures used to address infertility. These technologies help couples conceive when natural methods are unsuccessful. ART has advanced significantly, offering various options tailored to specific fertility challenges.

Intrauterine Insemination (IUI) IUI is a procedure where sperm is directly placed into the uterus, increasing the chances of fertilization by bringing sperm closer to the egg. It's often used for couples with mild male factor infertility, unexplained infertility, or cervical issues.

Procedure:

1. **Ovulation Monitoring**: The woman's menstrual cycle is monitored to determine the timing of ovulation. This can be done through ultrasound or ovulation predictor kits.
2. **Sperm Collection and Preparation**: A sperm sample is collected from the male partner or a donor. The sperm is then washed and concentrated to enhance motility.
3. **Insemination**: The prepared sperm is inserted into the uterus using a thin catheter during the woman's ovulation period.

In Vitro Fertilization (IVF) IVF is one of the most well-known and effective ART methods. It involves fertilizing an egg with sperm outside the body and then transferring the resulting embryo into the uterus.

Procedure:

1. **Ovarian Stimulation**: The woman takes hormonal medications to stimulate the ovaries to produce multiple eggs.
2. **Egg Retrieval**: Once the eggs are mature, they are retrieved from the ovaries using a minor surgical procedure under sedation.
3. **Fertilization**: The eggs are fertilized with sperm in a laboratory. This can be done using conventional IVF or intracytoplasmic sperm injection (ICSI) if there are severe male factor infertility issues.
4. **Embryo Culture**: The fertilized eggs (embryos) are cultured for several days in the lab.
5. **Embryo Transfer**: One or more healthy embryos are transferred into the woman's uterus. If successful, the embryo implants and begins to grow.

Intracytoplasmic Sperm Injection (ICSI) ICSI is a specialized form of IVF used primarily for severe male infertility. In this procedure, a single sperm is injected directly into an egg to facilitate fertilization.

Procedure:

1. **Egg Retrieval**: Eggs are retrieved from the ovaries as in the IVF process.
2. **Sperm Injection**: A single healthy sperm is selected and injected directly into each mature egg.
3. **Embryo Culture and Transfer**: The resulting embryos are cultured and transferred to the uterus, similar to standard IVF.

Third-Party Reproduction Third-party reproduction involves using donor eggs, sperm, or embryos, or a gestational carrier (surrogate) to achieve pregnancy.

- **Egg Donation**: Used when a woman's eggs are not viable due to age, premature ovarian failure, or genetic conditions. Donor eggs are fertilized with sperm, and the resulting embryos are transferred to the recipient's uterus.
- **Sperm Donation**: Used for severe male infertility, single women, or same-sex female couples. Donor sperm is used for IUI or IVF.
- **Embryo Donation**: Couples with surplus embryos from previous IVF cycles can donate them to other couples.

- **Gestational Surrogacy**: A gestational carrier (surrogate) carries the pregnancy for individuals or couples unable to do so. The embryo is created using the intended parents' or donors' gametes and transferred to the surrogate's uterus.

Success Rates and Considerations The success rates of ART procedures vary based on factors such as the woman's age, the cause of infertility, and the specific ART method used. Generally, younger women and those with fewer fertility issues have higher success rates. However, ART can be emotionally, physically, and financially demanding. It's important to have realistic expectations and consider counseling or support groups to navigate the process.

Ethical and Legal Considerations ART procedures can raise ethical and legal issues, particularly regarding third-party reproduction and the handling of embryos. It's crucial to understand the legal implications, such as parental rights and the regulation of donor and surrogate arrangements, which can vary by region. Consulting with legal and ethical experts can provide clarity and ensure informed decision-making.

The road to conception can be filled with excitement, hope, and challenges. Understanding when to stop birth control, timing intercourse, dealing with infertility, and exploring assisted reproductive technologies are critical steps in this journey. By making informed decisions and seeking appropriate medical guidance, you can enhance your chances of achieving a healthy and successful pregnancy.

Each couple's journey is unique, and it's essential to remain patient and open to various options. Support from healthcare providers, family, and friends can make a significant difference in navigating this path. Remember that advances in medical science continue to offer new solutions and hope for those facing fertility challenges.

Ultimately, the goal is to create a nurturing environment for conception and a healthy pregnancy. With the right information, support, and perseverance, the dream of becoming parents can become a reality.

Chapter 12: Early Pregnancy Signs and Symptoms

Recognizing Pregnancy Symptoms

The journey of pregnancy often begins with subtle signs that can be easily overlooked or mistaken for other conditions. Recognizing these early pregnancy symptoms can help you identify your pregnancy sooner, allowing you to start taking the necessary steps for a healthy gestation period. Understanding these signs can also help alleviate any anxiety or confusion you might experience during the early stages.

1. Missed Period

One of the most common and reliable early signs of pregnancy is a missed period. If your menstrual cycle is regular and you suddenly miss a period, it could be an indication that you are pregnant. However, missed periods can also be caused by stress, hormonal imbalances, or other medical conditions, so it is important to consider other symptoms as well.

2. Morning Sickness

Morning sickness, characterized by nausea and vomiting, typically starts around the sixth week of pregnancy but can begin as early as the fourth week. Despite its name, morning sickness can occur at any time of the day or night. It is caused by the rapid increase in hormones, particularly human chorionic gonadotropin (hCG) and estrogen. While it can be uncomfortable, morning sickness is generally a good sign that the pregnancy hormones are working properly.

3. Breast Changes

Early in pregnancy, hormonal changes can cause your breasts to become tender, swollen, or sore. Your nipples might also become more prominent, darker, and more sensitive. These changes are a result of increased blood flow and the preparation of your body for breastfeeding.

4. Fatigue

Feeling unusually tired is another common early pregnancy symptom. The surge in progesterone levels during the first trimester can make you feel more fatigued than usual. Additionally, your body is working hard to support the developing fetus, which can also contribute to increased tiredness.

5. Frequent Urination

In the early weeks of pregnancy, you may find yourself needing to urinate more frequently. This is due to the growing uterus pressing on your bladder, as well as increased blood flow to the kidneys, which results in more urine production.

6. Food Aversions and Cravings

Changes in your sense of taste and smell can occur early in pregnancy. You might develop aversions to certain foods or strong cravings for others. These changes are thought to be related to hormonal fluctuations.

7. Light Spotting or Cramping

Some women experience light spotting or cramping in the early stages of pregnancy, known as implantation bleeding. This occurs when the fertilized egg attaches to the lining of the uterus, usually around 10 to 14 days after conception. The bleeding is typically lighter than a normal period and lasts for a shorter duration.

8. Mood Swings

Hormonal changes during early pregnancy can affect your mood, causing you to feel more emotional or irritable than usual. Mood swings are a common symptom and can vary in intensity.

9. Elevated Basal Body Temperature

If you have been tracking your basal body temperature (BBT) to monitor ovulation, you might notice that your BBT remains elevated for more than two weeks after ovulation. This sustained rise in temperature can be an early indication of pregnancy.

10. Bloating and Constipation

Hormonal changes can also slow down your digestive system, leading to bloating and constipation. These symptoms can start early in pregnancy and may continue throughout the first trimester.

Recognizing these early pregnancy symptoms can help you identify a potential pregnancy, but it is important to confirm your pregnancy with a test and consultation with your healthcare provider.

Taking a Pregnancy Test

Once you suspect that you might be pregnant based on early symptoms, the next step is to take a pregnancy test. Pregnancy tests are designed to detect the presence of hCG, a hormone produced by the placenta shortly after the embryo attaches to the uterine lining. Here is a detailed guide on how to effectively take a pregnancy test and understand the results.

1. Types of Pregnancy Tests

There are two main types of pregnancy tests: home pregnancy tests (HPTs) and blood tests performed by a healthcare provider.

- **Home Pregnancy Tests (HPTs)**: These tests are available over-the-counter and can be easily done at home. They typically involve urinating on a test stick or dipping the stick into a urine sample. Results are usually displayed within a few minutes, indicating whether hCG is present in the urine.
- **Blood Tests**: These tests are performed at a healthcare facility and can detect lower levels of hCG than urine tests. There are two types of blood tests: qualitative hCG tests, which give a simple yes or no answer, and quantitative hCG tests, which measure the exact amount of hCG in the blood. Blood tests can confirm pregnancy earlier than urine tests and provide more detailed information about hCG levels.

2. Timing of the Test

For the most accurate results, it is best to wait until after you have missed your period to take a home pregnancy test. This is because hCG levels are typically high enough to be detected in urine by this time. Some sensitive tests can detect pregnancy a few days before a missed period, but testing too early can result in a false negative.

3. How to Take a Home Pregnancy Test

Follow these steps to ensure accurate results when taking a home pregnancy test:

- **Read the Instructions**: Each brand of HPT may have slightly different instructions, so it is important to read and follow them carefully.
- **Use the First Morning Urine**: For the most accurate results, use your first urine of the day, as it is usually more concentrated and has higher levels of hCG.
- **Collect the Urine**: Depending on the test, you may need to urinate directly onto the test stick or collect a urine sample in a clean container and dip the stick into it.
- **Wait for Results**: Place the test on a flat surface and wait for the amount of time specified in the instructions (usually a few minutes).
- **Interpret the Results**: Most tests will display lines, symbols, or digital readouts to indicate whether you are pregnant. A positive result usually shows two lines or a plus sign, while a negative result shows one line or a minus sign. Some digital tests will display "pregnant" or "not pregnant."

4. Confirming the Results

If you get a positive result on a home pregnancy test, it is important to confirm the pregnancy with your healthcare provider. They can perform a blood test to verify the results and provide you with more information about your pregnancy. If the home test is negative but you still suspect you are pregnant, wait a few days and retest or consult your healthcare provider for further evaluation.

Confirming Pregnancy with Your Doctor

After receiving a positive result on a home pregnancy test, the next step is to schedule an appointment with your healthcare provider to confirm the pregnancy. This initial visit is crucial for establishing a baseline of your health and ensuring the best possible care for you and your baby throughout the pregnancy.

1. Medical History and Physical Exam

During your first prenatal visit, your healthcare provider will review your medical history and perform a physical exam. They will ask about:

- Your menstrual cycle and the date of your last period
- Any previous pregnancies and their outcomes
- Your medical history, including chronic conditions, surgeries, and medications

- Family medical history, including genetic disorders
- Lifestyle factors, such as diet, exercise, and substance use

The physical exam may include checking your weight, blood pressure, and general health to establish a baseline for monitoring your pregnancy.

2. Confirmatory Tests

Your healthcare provider will perform additional tests to confirm the pregnancy and assess your health. These may include:

- **Blood Tests**: A blood test can confirm pregnancy by measuring hCG levels. Quantitative hCG tests can provide information about the exact amount of hCG in your blood, which can help estimate the gestational age of the pregnancy.
- **Ultrasound**: An ultrasound can provide visual confirmation of the pregnancy. During the early stages, a transvaginal ultrasound may be used to get a clear image of the uterus and confirm the presence of a gestational sac and, later, a fetal heartbeat.
- **Urine Tests**: Similar to home pregnancy tests, urine tests at the doctor's office can also detect hCG levels to confirm pregnancy.

3. Discussing Health and Lifestyle

Your healthcare provider will discuss various aspects of your health and lifestyle to ensure a healthy pregnancy. Topics may include:

- **Nutrition and Supplements**: Recommendations for a balanced diet and the importance of taking prenatal vitamins, including folic acid and iron.
- **Exercise**: Safe exercise routines to maintain health and fitness during pregnancy.
- **Avoiding Harmful Substances**: Guidance on avoiding alcohol, smoking, recreational drugs, and other harmful substances.
- **Managing Pre-existing Conditions**: How to manage chronic health conditions, such as diabetes or hypertension, during pregnancy.
- **Mental Health**: Addressing any concerns about stress, anxiety, or depression and discussing resources for mental health support.

4. Planning for Future Visits

Your healthcare provider will outline a schedule for future prenatal visits. Regular checkups are essential for monitoring the progress of your pregnancy and addressing any concerns that may arise. Typically, you will have monthly visits during the first and second trimesters, increasing in frequency as you approach your due date.

First Trimester Overview

The first trimester of pregnancy, spanning from week 1 to week 12, is a critical period for both you and your developing baby. During this time, significant changes occur in your body, and the foundations for your baby's growth and development are established.

1. Early Development

In the first few weeks of pregnancy, the fertilized egg implants itself in the lining of the uterus and begins to develop into an embryo. By the end of the first month, the embryo consists of three layers: the ectoderm, mesoderm, and endoderm, which will form the baby's organs and tissues. The neural tube, which will become the brain and spinal cord, also starts to form.

2. Hormonal Changes

The first trimester is marked by significant hormonal changes that support the pregnancy. The levels of hCG, progesterone, and estrogen rise rapidly. These hormones are responsible for many of the early pregnancy symptoms, such as nausea, breast tenderness, and fatigue.

3. Developmental Milestones

- **Weeks 4-5**: The heart begins to beat, and the basic structures of the brain, spinal cord, and major organs start to develop.
- **Weeks 6-7**: The embryo's facial features begin to form, including the eyes, nose, and mouth. The arms and legs start to bud.
- **Weeks 8-10**: The embryo is now referred to as a fetus. Major organs, such as the kidneys and liver, continue to develop. Fingers and toes start to form, and the fetus begins to move, although you won't feel it yet.
- **Weeks 11-12**: The fetus's vital organs are fully formed and will continue to mature throughout the pregnancy. The baby's external genitalia begin to show distinct male or female characteristics, though they may not be visible on an ultrasound yet.

4. Common Symptoms

- **Nausea and Vomiting**: Often referred to as morning sickness, these symptoms can occur at any time of the day and are usually most intense during the first trimester.
- **Fatigue**: Increased progesterone levels and the energy your body uses to support the pregnancy can cause significant tiredness.

- **Frequent Urination**: The growing uterus and increased blood flow to the pelvic area can lead to more frequent trips to the bathroom.
- **Breast Changes**: Hormonal changes can make your breasts feel tender, swollen, and more sensitive.
- **Mood Swings**: Hormonal fluctuations can affect your emotions, leading to mood swings.
- **Food Aversions and Cravings**: Changes in your sense of taste and smell can cause you to develop strong aversions or cravings for certain foods.

5. Important Health Practices

Maintaining good health practices during the first trimester is crucial for the well-being of both you and your baby. Here are some key practices to follow:

- **Balanced Diet**: Ensure you are eating a variety of nutrient-rich foods, including fruits, vegetables, whole grains, lean proteins, and dairy. Avoid foods that pose a risk of foodborne illness, such as raw or undercooked meats, unpasteurized dairy products, and certain types of fish high in mercury.
- **Hydration**: Drink plenty of water to stay hydrated, which helps support increased blood volume and amniotic fluid production.
- **Prenatal Vitamins**: Continue taking prenatal vitamins to ensure you and your baby receive

essential nutrients, including folic acid, iron, and calcium.

- **Exercise**: Engage in regular, moderate exercise, such as walking, swimming, or prenatal yoga, to maintain your fitness and manage stress.

- **Avoid Harmful Substances**: Refrain from smoking, drinking alcohol, and using recreational drugs. Limit caffeine intake and avoid exposure to toxic chemicals and radiation.

- **Rest and Relaxation**: Listen to your body and get plenty of rest. Practice stress-reducing techniques such as deep breathing, meditation, or gentle stretching.

6. Common Concerns and Complications

While most pregnancies progress without major issues, it is important to be aware of potential concerns and complications that can arise during the first trimester. Early detection and management can significantly improve outcomes.

- **Miscarriage**: The risk of miscarriage is highest during the first trimester. Symptoms may include heavy bleeding, severe cramping, and passing tissue. If you experience these symptoms, contact your healthcare provider immediately.

- **Ectopic Pregnancy**: An ectopic pregnancy occurs when the fertilized egg implants outside the uterus, usually in the fallopian tube. Symptoms include sharp abdominal pain, shoulder pain, and light to heavy vaginal bleeding. Ectopic pregnancy is a medical emergency and requires immediate attention.

- **Hyperemesis Gravidarum**: This condition is characterized by severe nausea and vomiting, leading to dehydration and weight loss. It is more intense than typical morning sickness and may require medical intervention.

- **Gestational Diabetes**: Though more commonly diagnosed later in pregnancy, some women may develop gestational diabetes early. It is important to manage blood sugar levels through diet, exercise, and, if necessary, medication.

7. Preparing for the Next Trimesters

The first trimester is just the beginning of your pregnancy journey. As you move into the second and third trimesters, you will experience new changes and milestones. It is important to continue attending regular prenatal visits, following a healthy lifestyle, and staying informed about your pregnancy.

By recognizing early pregnancy symptoms, confirming your pregnancy with a healthcare provider, and understanding what to expect during the first trimester, you are taking important steps towards a healthy and confident pregnancy. Each pregnancy is unique, and staying informed and proactive can help ensure the best possible outcomes for you and your baby.

The early stages of pregnancy are filled with a mix of excitement, anticipation, and, at times, uncertainty. By understanding and recognizing the early signs and symptoms of pregnancy, taking a reliable pregnancy test, confirming the pregnancy with your healthcare provider, and knowing what to expect during the first trimester, you can navigate this period with greater confidence and ease. Remember to take care of yourself, seek support when needed, and embrace the journey ahead with positivity and hope.

Chapter 13: Resources and Support

Embarking on the journey to parenthood is both exciting and overwhelming. One of the keys to navigating this period with confidence and peace of mind is having access to reliable resources and support systems. This chapter will provide you with a curated list of recommended books and websites, information on support groups and communities, guidance on finding a healthcare provider, and answers to frequently asked questions.

Recommended Books and Websites

Books

1. **What to Expect When You're Expecting by Heidi Murkoff** This classic book is a go-to guide for many expectant parents. It covers every stage of pregnancy, offering comprehensive information on physical changes, prenatal care, and what to expect during labor and delivery. The latest edition includes the most recent medical advice and reflects current trends in pregnancy and childbirth.

2. **The Mayo Clinic Guide to a Healthy Pregnancy by the Mayo Clinic** This guide is written by experts from the Mayo Clinic, providing evidence-based information on pregnancy. It covers everything from conception to post-delivery care, with detailed

chapters on fetal development, common pregnancy symptoms, and birthing options.

3. **Ina May's Guide to Childbirth by Ina May Gaskin** Ina May Gaskin, a renowned midwife, shares her wisdom and experience in this empowering book. It emphasizes natural childbirth and includes inspiring birth stories, practical advice, and information on the benefits of midwifery care.

4. **Expecting Better by Emily Oster** Emily Oster, an economist, examines the data behind common pregnancy advice. This book provides a rational approach to pregnancy, helping expectant parents make informed decisions based on statistical evidence rather than myths or misconceptions.

5. **The Pregnancy Encyclopedia by Paula Amato, M.D.** This encyclopedia is a comprehensive resource that covers all aspects of pregnancy. It includes detailed entries on various topics, illustrated guides, and expert advice from healthcare professionals.

Websites

1. **American Pregnancy Association** (www.americanpregnancy.org) This website offers a wealth of information on pregnancy, childbirth, and reproductive health. It includes articles on nutrition, prenatal care, labor and delivery, and postpartum care.

2. **The Bump** (www.thebump.com) The Bump provides personalized content and tools for expectant parents. It includes weekly updates on fetal development, checklists, and a community forum where parents can connect and share experiences.

3. **BabyCenter** (www.babycenter.com) BabyCenter is a comprehensive resource for pregnancy and parenting. It offers expert advice, interactive tools, and community support. The website covers a wide range of topics, including fertility, pregnancy symptoms, and baby care.

4. **Mayo Clinic Pregnancy** (www.mayoclinic.org/pregnancy) The Mayo Clinic's pregnancy section provides reliable, evidence-based information on all aspects of pregnancy. It includes articles on prenatal care, fetal development, and labor and delivery, written by healthcare professionals.

5. **What to Expect** (www.whattoexpect.com) This website, based on the popular book, offers week-by-week pregnancy updates, expert advice, and a supportive community for expectant parents. It covers a wide range of topics, including nutrition, exercise, and preparing for childbirth.

Online Support Groups

1. **BabyCenter Community** The BabyCenter Community is one of the largest online forums for expectant and new parents. It offers various groups based on due dates, specific interests, and parenting styles. Members can ask questions, share experiences, and offer support to one another.

2. **What to Expect Community** The What to Expect Community provides a platform for parents to connect, share advice, and support each other through pregnancy and parenting. The site includes groups based on due dates, geographic locations, and specific topics such as breastfeeding or sleep training.

3. **The Bump Community** The Bump Community offers a range of forums where expectant and new parents can discuss various topics related to pregnancy and parenting. The site also includes tools for tracking pregnancy progress and planning for baby's arrival.

4. **Reddit Parenting and Pregnancy Forums** Reddit hosts several active communities related to pregnancy and parenting, including r/pregnancy and r/parenting. These forums provide a platform for

parents to ask questions, share stories, and find support from others who are going through similar experiences.

In-Person Support Groups

1. **La Leche League International (www.llli.org)** La Leche League provides support and education for breastfeeding parents. The organization offers local support groups where parents can meet in person to share experiences, ask questions, and receive guidance from trained leaders.
2. **Meetup (www.meetup.com)** Meetup is a platform that helps people find and join local groups based on shared interests. Expectant and new parents can use Meetup to find local parenting groups, prenatal exercise classes, and other supportive communities.
3. **Hospital and Birth Center Support Groups** Many hospitals and birth centers offer support groups for expectant and new parents. These groups often include childbirth education classes, breastfeeding support, and postpartum support. Check with your healthcare provider or local hospital for available resources.

Specialized Support

1. **Postpartum Support International** (**www.postpartum.net**) Postpartum Support International provides resources and support for parents experiencing postpartum depression and other perinatal mood disorders. The organization offers online support groups, a helpline, and information on finding local resources.

2. **Resolve: The National Infertility Association** (**www.resolve.org**) Resolve offers support and education for individuals and couples experiencing infertility. The organization provides online support groups, educational resources, and information on finding local support groups and infertility specialists.

Finding a Healthcare Provider

Choosing the right healthcare provider is a crucial step in ensuring a healthy and confident pregnancy. Whether you prefer an obstetrician, a midwife, or a family doctor, it's important to find a provider who aligns with your values and needs. Here are some tips to help you find the right healthcare provider:

1. **Research Different Types of Providers**
   - **Obstetricians (OB-GYNs)**: Medical doctors who specialize in pregnancy, childbirth, and women's reproductive health.

- **Midwives**: Healthcare professionals who provide care during pregnancy, childbirth, and postpartum. They often emphasize natural childbirth and provide personalized, holistic care.
- **Family Doctors**: General practitioners who provide care for individuals and families across all ages, including prenatal and postpartum care.

2. **Consider Your Needs and Preferences**
   - Think about the type of birth experience you want (e.g., hospital birth, home birth, birthing center).
   - Consider any specific medical needs or conditions that may require specialized care.
   - Determine your preferences for prenatal care, such as the frequency of visits and the types of tests and screenings you are comfortable with.

3. **Ask for Recommendations**
   - Seek recommendations from friends, family, or colleagues who have had positive experiences with their healthcare providers.
   - Join local parenting groups or online forums to ask for recommendations from other expectant parents.

4. **Check Credentials and Experience**

- Ensure that the healthcare provider is licensed and board-certified in their specialty.
- Research their experience and any areas of specialization, such as high-risk pregnancies or natural childbirth.

5. **Schedule Consultations**

- Schedule consultations with potential providers to discuss your pregnancy plans and ask questions about their approach to prenatal care and childbirth.
- Use this opportunity to assess their communication style, bedside manner, and willingness to address your concerns.

6. **Evaluate Comfort and Trust**

- Choose a provider with whom you feel comfortable and can build a trusting relationship.
- Trust your instincts; if you feel uneasy or unsupported, it may be best to continue your search.

7. **Consider Hospital Affiliations**

- If you plan to give birth in a hospital, ensure that your healthcare provider has privileges at your preferred hospital.
- Research the hospital's policies, facilities, and support services, such as lactation consultants and postpartum care.

1. **When should I start taking prenatal vitamins?**
   - It is recommended to start taking prenatal vitamins at least three months before trying to conceive. This ensures that your body has adequate levels of essential nutrients, such as folic acid, which helps prevent neural tube defects in the baby.
2. **How often should I see my healthcare provider during pregnancy?**
   - Typically, you will have monthly prenatal visits during the first and second trimesters, bi-weekly visits during the third trimester, and weekly visits in the last month of pregnancy. Your healthcare provider may adjust the schedule based on your specific needs and any complications that arise.
3. **What should I avoid during pregnancy?**
   - Avoid smoking, alcohol, and recreational drugs. Limit caffeine intake to no more than 200 milligrams per day. Avoid raw or undercooked meat, fish high in mercury, unpasteurized dairy products, and certain types of soft cheeses.

Consult your healthcare provider for a comprehensive list of foods and substances to avoid.

4. **How can I manage morning sickness?**
   - Eat small, frequent meals throughout the day. Avoid foods and smells that trigger nausea. Stay hydrated and sip ginger tea or eat ginger candies. Rest and avoid sudden movements. If morning sickness is severe, consult your healthcare provider for additional treatments or medications.

5. **What are the signs of labor?**
   - Signs of labor include regular contractions that become more frequent and intense, lower back pain, cramping, the passing of the mucus plug, and the rupture of membranes (water breaking). If you experience any of these signs, contact your healthcare provider.

6. **Can I exercise during pregnancy?**
   - Yes, regular exercise is beneficial during pregnancy. Aim for at least 150 minutes of moderate-intensity exercise per week, such as walking, swimming, or prenatal yoga. Avoid high-impact activities, contact sports, and exercises that involve lying on your back after the first trimester. Always consult your healthcare provider before starting any new exercise routine.

7. **How can I prepare for breastfeeding?**

- Attend a breastfeeding class or workshop to learn about proper techniques and common challenges. Invest in a good quality breast pump and nursing bras. Create a comfortable breastfeeding space at home. Reach out to a lactation consultant for personalized support and guidance.

8. **What should I pack in my hospital bag?**

   - Essential items include your ID and insurance information, a birth plan, comfortable clothing, toiletries, a phone charger, snacks, and items for the baby such as clothes, diapers, and a blanket. Consider packing items for labor comfort, such as a birthing ball, music, and essential oils.

9. **How can I manage stress during pregnancy?**

   - Practice relaxation techniques such as deep breathing, meditation, and prenatal yoga. Maintain a healthy lifestyle with balanced nutrition and regular exercise. Seek support from your partner, family, and friends. If stress becomes overwhelming, consider speaking with a mental health professional.

10. **What should I do if I have a high-risk pregnancy?**

   - Follow your healthcare provider's recommendations closely. Attend all prenatal appointments and undergo any additional tests or screenings as advised. Maintain a healthy lifestyle and avoid any activities or substances that could

increase risk. Seek support from specialists, such
as a maternal-fetal medicine doctor, if needed.

Access to reliable resources and support is crucial for a
healthy and confident pregnancy journey. By leveraging
the recommended books, websites, and support groups, and
by finding a trusted healthcare provider, you can ensure
that you are well-prepared for the challenges and joys of
pregnancy. Remember, every pregnancy is unique, and it's
important to stay informed, ask questions, and seek support
when needed. Congratulations on your pregnancy, and we
wish you a smooth and joyful journey to parenthood.

Conclusion

Final Thoughts and Encouragement

As you embark on the incredible journey of pregnancy, it's important to recognize the profound impact this period will have on your life. Pregnancy is not just a physical process but a transformative experience that reshapes your emotional and mental landscape. Throughout this book, we've aimed to equip you with the knowledge and tools needed to navigate this journey with confidence and grace.

Understanding the intricacies of preconception health, the importance of lifestyle adjustments, and the significance of mental and emotional preparation are all critical components of a healthy and fulfilling pregnancy. Each chapter has been designed to provide you with comprehensive information and practical advice, helping you make informed decisions every step of the way.

Pregnancy is a unique experience for every individual and couple. While the journey may have its challenges, it's also filled with moments of joy, anticipation, and deep connection. As you move forward, remember that it's okay to seek help, ask questions, and lean on your support network. Your healthcare providers, family, and friends are invaluable resources, ready to support you through this life-changing process.

It's also essential to be kind to yourself. The journey to parenthood is a marathon, not a sprint. There will be days of excitement and days of uncertainty, but each step brings you closer to meeting your baby. Celebrate the small victories, acknowledge your efforts, and trust in your ability to handle whatever comes your way.

Looking Forward to the Journey Ahead

Looking ahead, the road to parenthood is filled with many milestones. From the moment you first suspect you might be pregnant, through the trimesters, to the birth of your child, each phase offers new experiences and challenges. It's crucial to stay informed and proactive, continually learning and adapting as your pregnancy progresses.

First Trimester: This initial stage is often marked by excitement and significant physical changes. It's a time to establish healthy habits, attend regular prenatal checkups, and begin preparing for the months ahead. Morning sickness, fatigue, and other early pregnancy symptoms can be managed with proper care and attention to your body's needs.

Second Trimester: Often referred to as the "golden period" of pregnancy, the second trimester typically brings relief from early symptoms and a surge in energy. It's an excellent time to start planning for your baby's arrival, including setting up the nursery, attending childbirth classes, and continuing to monitor your health and well-being.

Third Trimester: As you approach the final stages of pregnancy, focus on preparing for labor and delivery. Attend prenatal appointments regularly, discuss your birth plan with your healthcare provider, and ensure you have everything ready for your baby's arrival. It's also a time to focus on rest and self-care, as your body will need to conserve energy for the upcoming birth.

Labor and Delivery: This stage can be both exhilarating and challenging. Having a well-thought-out birth plan, understanding your pain management options, and knowing what to expect during labor can help ease anxiety and ensure a smoother experience. Trust in your body's ability to give birth and lean on your support team for encouragement and assistance.

Postpartum Period: The journey doesn't end with the birth of your baby. The postpartum period is a critical time for recovery and adjustment. Focus on your physical recovery, emotional well-being, and adapting to the new demands of parenthood. Seek support from healthcare providers, family, and friends to navigate this transition successfully.

Throughout this journey, it's important to stay connected with your partner, communicate openly about your experiences, and support each other. Building a strong partnership will not only help you during pregnancy but also lay a solid foundation for your parenting journey.

Acknowledgements

Creating this book has been a labor of love, and it wouldn't have been possible without the contributions and support of many individuals. We extend our deepest gratitude to everyone who played a part in bringing this comprehensive guide to life.

First and foremost, we would like to thank the healthcare professionals who generously shared their expertise and insights. Their contributions have been invaluable in ensuring that the information presented is accurate, relevant, and up-to-date.

We are also immensely grateful to the many parents who shared their personal experiences and stories. Their openness and honesty have added a rich, human element to this book, making it relatable and engaging for our readers. Your journeys inspire and remind us of the unique and diverse paths to parenthood.

Our appreciation goes to the team of editors, designers, and publishers who have worked tirelessly to bring this book to fruition. Your dedication, creativity, and attention to detail have made this project a success. Thank you for your hard work and commitment to excellence.

A heartfelt thank you to our families and friends for their unwavering support and encouragement throughout this process. Your belief in this project and your understanding of the countless hours invested have been a source of strength and motivation.

Lastly, we extend our deepest gratitude to you, the reader. Your decision to embark on this journey and seek out knowledge and guidance is commendable. We hope that this book serves as a valuable resource, providing you with the confidence and support you need to navigate pregnancy and parenthood.

In conclusion, the journey to parenthood is one of the most profound and transformative experiences in life. By taking proactive steps, seeking support, and staying informed, you are setting the stage for a healthy and fulfilling pregnancy. Embrace the journey with an open heart, trust in your abilities, and know that you are not alone. Congratulations on this incredible journey, and we wish you all the best as you prepare to welcome your new baby into the world.

I HAVE A REQUEST

Dear Reader,

Thank you for your purchase! We hope you enjoyed the book. We would greatly appreciate it if you could leave an honest review.

Your honest feedback is essential for our growth and helps us understand what you value most. By sharing your thoughts, you not only help other readers make informed choices but also increase the visibility of this book.

Your words can inspire and guide others, creating a community built on shared insights and connections. Let's celebrate meaningful communication and the beauty of heartfelt expressions together.

Thank you!

www.ingramcontent.com/pod-product-compliance
Lightning Source LLC
Chambersburg PA
CBHW051611250726
48653CB00004BA/1446